Guidebook for a Healthy Lifestyle:
Wellness and You

Reverend Albert Wingfield

CTS Family Press
Fort Wayne, Indiana

Library of Congress Card Catalog Number: 2007929858

ISBN 978-1-930260-16-0

Dedication

This book is dedicated to my wife, Marge, who has made reading food labels, preparing proper foods, and putting proper portions on our table a way of life and an adventure with me to maintain a spiritual and physical wellness lifestyle.

To our children and grandchildren, who are very much aware of the importance of wellness, both spiritual and physical, from birth to the time we become senior citizens.

To Linda (Wingfield) Krohn, teacher and one who cares about children and her family, who has helped with and co-written part of this book.

To Michelle Wilkinson, who has used her knowledge as a practicing physician's assistant and her commitment to wellness to support this book.

To all of the Concordia Theological Seminary students and staff who have worked hard to prove what the book advocates: If you want to be physically well, you need to exercise and eat properly.

To Zion Lutheran Church, Corunna, Indiana, which has supported a spiritual and physical wellness program, especially Dave and Carol Swogger, Sandy and Dave Bartolin, Charlie and Linda Martz, Carolyn Martz and her late husband Don Martz, and Jake and Sally Waltenburg, who were very instrumental in getting the wellness ministry started.

To Louise "Aunt Kit" Hill and her family, especially daughter Colleen Mays and her husband Doug, who know what wellness means to a loved one.

And finally, to my lifetime friends, Johnny and Sissy Farchman, Richard Hoffman, and Jimmy and Ima Fay Pelton. These two families know the real meaning of wellness and the importance of loving care. Johnny, Jimmy, and Richard will always remember the midnight run for wellness.

Al Wingfield

Table of Contents

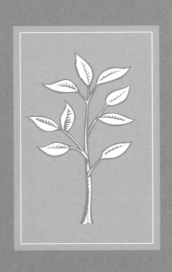

Introduction

It Is Worth Your Life

This is a true story about a significant event in my life. I want to use the experience to urge you, no matter whether you are male or female, to listen to your body. It may be trying to tell you something that could save your life. I also want to encourage you to use this *Guidebook for a Healthy Lifestyle* as a tool. If you follow the guidelines of this book, it will help you have a healthy and fit body and keep it that way.

Now my story. I enjoyed a normal childhood. I lived on a farm and enjoyed all the good things of growing up. I have a younger brother and many cousins. There were no major illnesses in the family as we grew up. In high school I played basketball and football and kept in good physical condition. Immediately after high school I entered the military service and spent five years in the U.S. Navy during the Korean conflict (that dates me).

Shortly after enlisting in the Navy, I married my high school sweetheart, Marge. We have been blessed with six children and 18 grandchildren and will celebrate 55 years of marriage in 2008. With my degree in elementary and secondary education, we have traveled all over the United States and to Japan and Hong Kong serving The Lutheran Church–Missouri Synod. I taught physical education and coached for many years, and I have always been healthy.

With a keen interest in aerobics and cardiovascular health I had read many of Dr. Ken Cooper's books on health. His team visited the Concordia Theological Seminary campus in Fort Wayne, Indiana, to train and certify aerobic instructors. After training with his team, I became an aerobic instructor. I have worked with individuals and taught classes since the 1980s.

In April of 2001, at 67 years of age, I felt good, ran on our treadmill five days a week, and carried a solid 204 pounds on my 5'10" frame. During the first part of the month I was dealing with a cold, so I stopped exercising for a few days. Then I started back on my exercise routine of walking a 15-minute mile for 60 minutes.

About halfway through the first day back, I felt a slight, but different, burning sensation in the upper right part of my chest. However, I finished the exercise with no pain and no problems. The next day I had the same slight sensation again. I thought it was probably cilia in my lungs that had been irritated from the cold.

So I had an X-ray, which showed my lungs were clear and everything was normal. My doctor said, "Al, why don't you do a treadmill test?" We scheduled the test to check my heart, and, again, I had a little of the same sensation but it was very slight. The treadmill test showed no problem.

I asked the doctor how we could know for sure if I had any blood flow blockage in my heart. He replied, "We will need to catheterize you." My reply was, "No way, that is invasive!"

The procedure entails inserting a tiny catheter into an artery in the groin. The catheter has the ability to give a clear picture of blood flow in all of the vessels. In other words, any plaque or mal-function in the artery is displayed on a screen, which gives a clear picture of the artery being catheterized. The doctor laughed, and I got up and started to leave.

As I moved to go out the door, the doctor said, "Al, as active as you are, let's go ahead and perform the catheterization. Then we will know for sure, without a doubt. If there is any blockage we could angioplasty it at the time of catheterization."

I thought a moment and then asked when we could do this. His reply was, "Tomorrow we have an opening." That would be Friday, April 20, 2001.

I did not tell Marge, my wife, that I was going to be catheterized. I told her I was just having some tests, and she dropped me off at the hospital. The procedure lasted 30 minutes, and the attendants talked and visited while the procedure was going on. When it was finished, they told me to get dressed, and I called Marge to pick me up.

As I sat waiting, my doctor came in and sat down beside me. I thought he looked distressed. He said, "Al, I do not know how to tell you this, but you are a walking time bomb. Your three major arteries are 95% blocked." My response was, "Well, Doctor, you can angioplasty it out." His reply was, "No."

I asked him about medication. He looked at me and said in a matter of fact way, "You are scheduled for open-heart surgery on Monday, April 23. Be at the hospital on Monday at 6:00 a.m."

I was angry, wondering how this could happen to me. I had always tried to take care of myself by eating right, exercising, and getting yearly routine physicals. I said, "Well, no more exercise for me." He smiled and said, "If you had not exercised, you would be dead." Then he showed me the blockage in my arteries and how new blood paths had formed as a result of my exercise routine to compensate for the blockage. I could see the large arteries were almost completely blocked.

Pastor gave me communion. My family was by my side. As many of you who have had surgery know, it is a long ride from the "holding area" to the operating room. I never thought about not making it through. But I knew that if I didn't make it through, I would wake up in heaven.

Six hours later, I became aware of Rebecca, my daughter, and Phil, my son, standing over my bed. I stuck my tongue out at

Rebecca and knew that I was among the living. Four days later I was home and a week later I was in rehabilitation.

The rehabilitation changed my lifestyle and more importantly, how much fat I consume each day. That is the main reason for this *Guidebook for a Healthy Lifestyle.*

I learned very quickly that my blockage in the arteries came as a result of too much fat in my diet. With exercise and the proper fat intake and other eating and lifestyle changes, I knew I could reverse what could have been disaster for me — and what can be disaster for you. A year after my surgery I am at my proper weight of 164 pounds, and I exercise for 60 minutes six to seven days a week.

I hope this book will help you listen to your body and respond to what the Lord says, "Take care of your body."

Al Wingfield

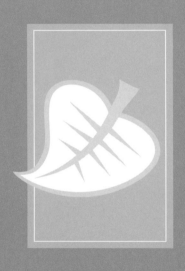

CHAPTER ONE

Why All the Hype about Wellness?

Listen to the radio, tune in to the television, read any newspaper or magazine. Before very long wellness and the family and what kind of program is needed to get Americans back into wellness lifestyle will be discussed. Statistics point to the fact that 61% of Americans are overweight.

Health insurance continues to escalate, putting many employers into a position where they are no longer able to provide a health plan that many employees can afford.

We all know that we live in a high tech, high stress world — a world where job, school, sports, and social demands are impacting our children, youth, married couples, families, and senior citizens. Yet, we are also blessed to live in a time when there is an abundance of food and medicines to combat all kinds of diseases. We have excellent medical facilities and highly skilled medical personnel.

However, the global world and the technical information society have placed some real challenges on how individuals and families live and function in our world today. Wellness from cradle to grave has become something that we must strive to achieve. We must use the tools available to us to identify our personal wellness plan and learn to implement a plan for us and those who depend on us. The goal of this book is to help people of all ages and in all walks of life have a wellness plan that fits their needs at this particular time in life.

As Christians, we know that we start our wellness plan with the spiritual, our relationship with God through Jesus Christ our personal Savior. We belong to Him, both physically and spiritually. As members of His divine family our goal is total wellness.

Spiritual wellness means spiritual food. In a time when God's Word should have the highest priority in our lives, we are told there is a decline in church and Sunday School attendance in all mainline congregations.

In our past the church was the focal point of family life — adult Bible class, Sunday School, Vacation Bible School, youth groups, and men's and women's Christian organizations. All of these activities revolved around the church. Now the family is fragmented. In the average family (if there is a family you can call average) both Mom and Dad work, and the children are placed in day care at a very tender age. The day care provider has much more influence over the children than do the parents. The families vie for quality time as the children move into elementary school life, and time becomes more hectic with work, school sports, church activities, etc.

A well planned spiritual time needs to take place as part of a wellness lifestyle. The adult caregiver/caregivers (many today facing these challenges alone) have to make healthy lifestyle plans.

A spiritual, healthy lifestyle means being into the Word of God on a regular basis. Romans 10:17 tells us, "So then faith cometh by hearing and hearing by the Word of God." II Timothy 3:16 informs us that, "All Scripture is God breathed and is useful for teaching, rebuking, correcting, and training in righteousness so that the man of God may be thoroughly equipped for every good work."

We read in Matthew 19:14, "Jesus said, 'Let the little children come to Me and do not hinder them, for the kingdom of heaven belongs to such as these.'" God provides His Holy Word, pastors, and teachers who work in our churches and schools. He expects the adult caregiver to head up the spiritual, healthy lifestyle in the home. Therefore, we are expected to have family devotions. We are expected to attend Bible class, Sunday School, church services, and other support programs for spiritual growth and food for all of

God's children, church workers and their families, and congregation members and their families.

When we consider wellness and a healthy lifestyle, we need to look at our family structure. In my book, *Marriage Is for Life, No Broken Promises, No Shattered Dreams*, I point out the most important factors for a child to succeed. These factors include coming from a two-parent family where by example the parents show their love for each other and their children. The children are taught a work ethic, and they have a high degree of self-confidence. This is the result of the home environment which was nurtured by both parents. They are well disciplined and understand consequences and accountability. This is also the result of two parents who support each other in love and discipline.

Then comes the time in one's life when the children are grown, and retirement is around the corner. We have put on a few pounds, and it is at this point in our lives that we need to sit back and take stock. Can you and your spouse answer "yes" to the following questions?

- Do you have a retirement plan that protects both of you in case of illness or death?

- Do you have a living will and have you made your funeral arrangements?

- Do you have a complete physical every year and do you have a good talking relationship with your doctor and care providers?

- Are both of you in an exercise program that meets your needs at this particular time in your lives?

- What are your plans when you retire? If both of you work, have you discussed this, and do you have a real plan of action in place?

- What about finances: Will you be covered by health insurance after you retire? Is Social

Security a part of your retirement or have you opted out of Social Security because you are considered self-employed and you have that option? Are you sure you have the financial protection you need?

- What about church? If you are a church worker, pastor, teacher, or whatever your calling has been (such as business man, housewife, farmer, or office worker), your church and your community still need you.

God has placed you in His world at a unique time in the history of His church, a time when He has provided us with technology and medical treatment that has made it possible for men and women and their families to live longer.

Reading and using this *Guidebook for a Healthy Lifestyle* will aid in a wellness plan that can help improve your quality of life.

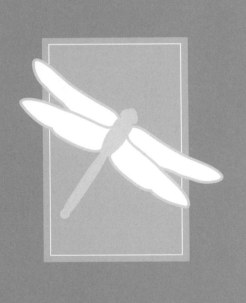

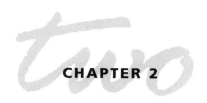

CHAPTER 2

Wellness and the Family: The Formative Years

Linda Wingfield Krohn, an educator and mother of four, has worked with and taught children at different formative levels in their lives. Linda is one who is vitally concerned about the family and wellness. She shares these ideas about children's formative years, birth through teens, and how families can put their children on the road to a lifelong healthy lifestyle:

When asked to contribute my thoughts on a wellness plan for a family centering on the needs of children and youth, I first wanted to define wellness, especially as it relates to young people. The dictionary gives such insight, and here are some small excerpts found under the word "wellness":

- In good health
- To distinguish oneself
- With care or completeness
- Heartily
- With reason
- In good manner
- Good conduct
- Of good family
- Wisely

These words give a great picture of the definition of "wellness."

Wellness can be defined as being in a healthy place — spiritually, physically, intellectually, creatively, and emotionally. This healthy place allows a person to meet the many trials and joys of this earthly life.

What an awesome challenge and responsibility we, as parents, face as we strive to bring this gift to our children. As a mom, it is my prayer that my children will carry a knowledge and practice of wellness into their adult life, so that they may serve God and others while here on earth.

How steadfast and committed we, as parents and authorities, must be to bring this gift of wellness to children. We are told in the Bible that the devil is like a lion prowling around, seeking to devour us; he knows our weaknesses and preys upon them. Young people today are faced with so much pressure and temptation that having a healthy, balanced life is a difficult thing to possess. Problems with school, peers, money, sports, technology, health, and so much more can make life seem like it's just too much at times.

Almost every aspect of our lives (even good things like eating) can be a problem when there is no balance. Just the pace alone of this modern world brings a stress that is challenging for all of us to face. But as mentioned earlier in this book, His Word provides us with a foundation and security so that we can meet these challenges and that our life on this earth may be one of joy and wellness.

One of the greatest challenges adults face is really "hearing" our young people. We are often too busy and facing our own difficulties to listen well to the young people who are put in our care. Here are some thoughts from young people I deeply respect.

A young adult had this to say:

> Wellness is a healthy lifestyle, spiritually and physically. It is a clear awareness of right and wrong and a sharp conscience. (Consciences can become dulled and insensitive if unused.) It is closeness to God with a healthy body.

Challenges that face young adult "wellness" are addictions (alcohol, drugs), immoral lifestyles (sex, language, and violence), peer pressure, unhealthy foods, and the world.

Habits that help a young adult be "well" are eating healthily (limit sweet foods and choose fruits, vegetables, protein, juices, milk), attending church weekly, reading the Bible with devotions daily, practicing abstinence, drinking alcohol moderately (if over 21), not smoking addictively, and practicing good relationships with friends and family.

A teenager had this to say:

Wellness is a state of balance in a person's life, where one is able to be content with his/her life. It is when one is able to deal with daily struggles in a positive way and to be thankful; a sense of peace.

Challenges that face teenage "wellness" are not having a continuous daily relationship with God, weight, sense of ongoing failure, trying to "look good" and "please the crowd," time and busyness, pressure to do good/be perfect, work (school, job), laziness, gradual "opening" to language, bad morals (in general), and uncontrolled activities such as food intake.

Habits that help a teenager to be "well" are getting enough sleep, eating healthily and exercising, applying skills and talents in the best possible way, always finding something to be thankful and grateful for, looking past mistakes and failures, using time wisely, not worrying about self but thinking about how you can help and affect somebody else, and hard work.

A pre-adolescent had this to say:

Wellness is eating reasonable amounts, exercising daily, eating fruits and vegetables, eating good food, washing hands, watching for germy things, not too much time with electronics, and exercising your brain with reading.

Challenges that face teenage "wellness" are the way you think you have to look, being too busy, and feeling pressure from other people.

Habits that help a teenager to be "well" are exercising, eating enough/not too much, and studying hard.

A young child had this to say:

Being healthy is being strong. A strong person believes in God. Being healthy is a person who eats fruit, covers mouth (good habits), doesn't smoke, reads, runs, does his/her best work, and doesn't sit around and watch TV.

Based on the insights and observations of these and many other young people, wellness is the state of being balanced spiritually, physically, intellectually, creatively, and emotionally. A wellness plan for a family is one that addresses all of these needs and strives to keep them all in balance. Habits and routines that are established and followed through is one foundation children and adults need in order to live a healthy and balanced life.

We actually all crave routine and habits. Our body and mind can move forward through stress and struggle when we are in a place with good habits and routines established in our lives. An integral part of the development of any habit or routine is accountability. Holding one another accountable says "I love you" even if it doesn't feel that way. Children may often say "I don't care" when they are held accountable, but they know inside that someone cared enough to discipline and love them. The highest level of accountability is when our children are motivated out of love and a desire to serve our Heavenly Father.

A challenge that all of us face is being so verbal (empty words) that children no longer hold our words as "the truth." It is following through that counts. Regardless of the situation, following through says "I love you" and "I care." It is important for us as parents to choose words wisely so we are consistent and the accountability expectation is consistent, as well. Taking the time to teach habits, live by them, and practice accountability are essential to establishing a wellness plan for families.

This leads to another foundation of wellness: communication. Young people are faced with so much technology (television, computers, iPods, and so forth), leaving so little time at the table eating together or in a kitchen or garage working side by side with Mom or Dad, that they have not learned the art of conversing and working well with others. A friend of mine recently commented on the young people who walk around with their hoods up and eyes down. We discussed how what is really being said is "I am insecure and not comfortable with who I am."

After many years of working with and observing young people, those who seem to be in a healthier place are those who can discuss and debate the struggles and sins of daily life. When we can be honest about our sins and difficulties, it makes life easier to deal with. We often discover that others have the same or similar struggles, and we no longer feel that we are the only ones who think or struggle with a temptation or sin and then feel a guilt that shouldn't be there. Teaching children to look others in the eye, to greet and acknowledge one another, and to be able to converse and share with others is an important foundation of wellness.

Another foundation of wellness is selflessness. "It's not all about you" is an important attitude that young people and adults alike need to be reminded of and strive to live by. Our sinful nature causes us too often to think of ourselves first. Healthy people carry with them a sense of service and a "giving" attitude that is healthy and positive.

The ultimate gift of selflessness was Jesus' gift for us. When we are in His Word, we learn this love of Jesus Christ, which was so great that He suffered and died on the cross. With this sacrifice comes the gift of forgiveness.

Being able to forgive ourselves and to forgive others is essential to any wellness plan. We all daily sin much and make many mistakes. Forgiveness allows us to move forward, striving to do our best, but knowing that His mercy covers us no matter how big our failure.

Being spiritually healthy is being in His Word. Worshiping with our children on a regular basis is a fundamental need. A gift that my mom and dad brought to our family was the simple practice of having devotions at the supper table together. I have many special memories of discussion, laughter, learning, and, yes, even arguing. I am amazed now at the discussions my own family has as we sit together around the table.

Busy schedules that prevent the coming together of families for eating and sharing their day with one another is a weapon Satan has used mightily in our world today. The simple habit of coming together, eating, and having devotions is a golden opportunity for families.

Being in His Word and receiving the Sacrament is important for spiritual healthiness, as well. Regular worship, coming together for family devotions, and being forgiving to one another are three habits that allow a family to be spiritually healthy.

Being physically healthy is maintaining balance in the core areas of eating, exercising, and sleeping. It sounds so simple, but this is difficult to accomplish with our busy overscheduled lives.

One simple plan for physical health is to focus on exercising rather than eating. Girls, especially, over-focus on food, which causes an imbalance in their diet. The simple plan of eating healthy meals with snacks and not to forbid certain foods (like desserts) is important. People who have an exercise plan and stick with it (even if imperfectly) don't think about food so much, and by that simple focus are more successful in keeping these areas of food and exercise in balance.

The exercising of our intellect through the love of reading, music, and lifelong learning is an important aspect of being well also. Children and young adults who appreciate and cultivate these three gifts that God has given us have a healthier and more positive spirit.

Being well in the area of creativity is one that is often over-looked. Allowing the time and enjoyment of God's many gifts to us is important and helps keep us well. Whether it's baking, hiking, painting, playing an instrument, reading, or planting a garden, being creative with our hands is important. Our Heavenly Father is our Creator. Our hands to create and serve Him are a natural and needed response.

Being emotionally healthy is accomplished by bringing the physical, spiritual, intellectual, and creative together so that one can meet the daily joys and stress of life. The fruits of the Spirit are then able to be reflected and shared with those around us in an imperfect, but blessed way.

The gifts of the Spirit are love, joy, peace, patience, kindness, goodness, faithfulness, gentleness, and self-control. It is my prayer that we as parents and authorities teach and nurture wellness in our young people so they can go forth and serve Him with their many gifts.

Healthy Balance

Make a plan ←——→ Be flexible

Be firm ←——→ Be loving

Be determined ←——→ Be understanding

Strive for your best ←——→ Learn from failures

Be generous ←——→ Be thrifty

Be tenacious ←——→ Be gentle

Hold firm ←——→ Let it go

Speak ←——→ Listen

Do for others ←——→ Take care of yourself

Live by the law ←——→ Live in grace

Fruits of the Spirit

love, joy, peace, patience,
kindness, goodness, faithfulness,
gentleness, and self-control

WELLNESS
is
being

spiritually
physically
intellectually
creatively
emotionally

in
balance

habits/routines
accountability
communication
selflessness
forgiveness

His Word

Healthy Attitudes

- Pray.
- Be of concern, not worry.
- Believe in yourself.
- Be able to step into one another's shoes.
- Mistakes are amazing when we learn from them.
- Don't make it bigger than it is.
- Be wise with God's gift of time.
- Be confident; you can do it.
- Be content.
- Let it go; forgive one another.

Healthy Exercise

- Make a plan.
- Incorporate exercise into daily life.
- Stay on track if you miss a day.
- Give yourself a day of rest.
- Choose a time that works for your body.
- Make yourself accountable.
- Make small changes and stick to them.
- Educate yourself.
- Exercise your body and brain.
- Do what you love.

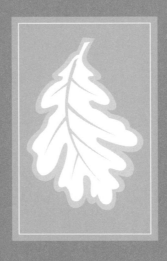

CHAPTER 3

Wellness and Our Senior Citizens

To help us respond to the challenges in our wellness plan from cradle to grave, the following information is provided by Michelle Wilkinson, P.A., member of the American Academy of Physician's Assistants and Indiana Academy of Physician's Assistants. She offers a wealth of information about good lifestyle choices and preventive medicine for our senior citizens:

As we consider those in their 60s and 70s, these were considered the golden years, but in the last decade, with rising health care costs and the risks of being uninsured or underinsured, many seniors are continuing to work. That magical age of 65 brings us to screenings for abdominal aortic aneurysm and osteoporosis and pneumonia vaccine.

As we look beyond the 70s, the health maintenance exam is still important. We may not be preventing disease processes, but keeping a close eye on them not only creates quantity of life but quality of life. We also must prepare patients for the end of life — finding out what their final wishes are and how much medical support they would like.

Studies have proven time and time again the value of preventive medicine. Thus far we have discussed from the cradle to middle age. Now we need to look at the other spectrum of life — those considered seniors.

There have been great strides in the Medicare program over the last few years, namely, with the privatization of the previously government-run program. That change has given the decision making to private companies that have been working with the health care industry for years, allowing each health care dollar to be spent more efficiently. With any change there are always bumps in the road, but these companies know that prevention is the key at any age and at any time. The government realized that traditional insurance offers much more in the way of preventive medicine, and this is truly the way to provide the absolute best health care for perhaps the largest group of people who take advantage of health benefits.

Prevention

Prevention really is the best medicine! The most important risk factor is family history. A little knowledge about your immediate family members can provide a directed and more purposeful health plan. It gives your health care provider a route to take.

But your own health history is also important. It is important to know your chronic illnesses, if any; the medications you are taking; any previous surgeries; and pertinent social history, for example, smoking history or excess alcohol consumption.

You must feel comfortable talking to your health care provider, because you may have to discuss sensitive topics and reveal information that may be embarrassing otherwise. Personalities do clash, and doctors, nurses, etc. are human; therefore, it is important that you find a provider you are able to talk with freely. Always know that anything you discuss with a health care professional is confidential and will not leave the exam room.

Once you have your family history list made, you must also make a list of your current medications. Oftentimes people are seeing several different health care providers, and it is important that they all have a copy of current medications, including vitamins and herbal supplements. Some medications will interact with others and may interact with certain vitamins. You may be putting yourself at risk by not disclosing all medication information.

The first step in getting your preventive schedule started is with your doctor. So many of us are generally healthy, and perhaps we have not been to the doctor for ten years or more. Although it is often thought that this is a good thing, in the eyes of the medical community and the insurance companies this is quite possibly one of the worst things that can happen. When we look at the number one cause of death in adults over 65 — heart disease — it is in most cases preventable.

Heart disease is associated with or caused by diabetes, high blood pressure, smoking, improper diet, and lack of exercise. Heart disease is not something that is a killer overnight; it takes years to see the final effects of all of these risk factors.

A thorough physical exam by your physician allows you time to review your past medical history, make sure you are up to date with shots (no they are not just for kids any more), and talk about any screening exams that may be necessary.

If we consider the top ten causes of death in people over 65, we see why the current recommendations are in effect:

- Heart Disease
- Cancer
- Cerebrovascular Accident (stroke)
- Chronic Obstructive Pulmonary Disease (COPD)
- Pneumonia
- Diabetes
- Accidents
- Septicemia
- Nephritis (kidney disease)
- Alzheimer's Disease

The Current Recommendations

Let's take a look at the current recommendations for the most common preventable or controllable chronic illnesses.

Heart Disease: Cardiovascular recommendations have come under great scrutiny as of late, mainly due to the sharp rise in cardiovascular disease in the last two to three decades, especially in women. The American Heart Association is promoting a healthy lifestyle and risk reduction by having routine cholesterol and blood pressure screenings, maintaining proper weight, better food habits, exercise, and smoking cessation. We are not just talking about reducing the risk of heart attack but also stroke and sudden cardiac death.

High cholesterol, high blood pressure, and diabetes are direct risk factors for heart disease. Tight control of these direct risk factors for heart disease will improve the outcome dramatically.

Abdominal aortic aneurysm screening is recommended for men aged 65-75 who have smoked. For men who have never smoked and women the screening is not recommended unless there is a family history.

Cancer: Breast cancer is the second leading cause of death in women. Early detection is the key. It is recommended that all women over age 40 get a yearly mammogram; a baseline mammogram should be obtained between the ages of 35-39. Women should be particularly cautious if they have any of the following risk factors:

- Had breast cancer in the past.
- Have a family history of breast cancer (mother, sister, daughter, or two or more close relatives who have had breast cancer).
- Had a first baby after age 30.
- Have never had a baby.

- Used hormone replacement therapy (HRT) for a long period of time after menopause.

- Have two or more alcoholic drinks every day.

- Are overweight or obese, especially with weight gained during adulthood.

- Don't exercise.

- Are a Jew of Eastern European descent (an Ashkenazi Jew).

The recent Women's Health Initiative study has dramatically changed how we treat menopause, and we have discovered that HRT actually is counterproductive and significantly increases the risk of breast cancer. The current recommendation is not to start HRT, and if absolutely necessary, to use the lowest dose possible for the shortest amount of time.

For cervical and vaginal cancer, a Pap test is recommended every two years for women with no risk factors. With additional risk factors or an abnormal Pap test within the last three years, the recommendation is a Pap test every year. Those additional risk factors include whether you:

- Have had an abnormal Pap test.

- Have had cancer in the past.

- Have been infected with the Human Papillomavirus (HPV).

- Began having sex before age 16.

- Have had many sexual partners.

- Have a mother who took DES (diethylstilbestrol), a hormonal drug, when she was pregnant with you.

- Have a diet that is low in fruits and vegetables.

- Are overweight or obese.

- Have had many full-term pregnancies.

A new quadravelent vaccine for HPV, which is the leading cause of cervical cancer, was released in 2006. This vaccine may dramatically decrease the rate of cervical cancer, but at this time the vaccine is too new to predict the final results. The currently recommended age for the vaccine is starting at age nine; booster vaccine ages are not known yet.

Colorectal cancer screening is recommended for both men and women over age 50. For most people, this is the most dreaded screening, but if, like all of the other cancers, it is detected, early treatment succession rates are nearly 100%.

There are several tests that can be used to detect possible colorectal cancer other than the colonoscopy. Fecal occult blood testing, barium enema, and flexible sigmoidoscopy are all alternatives to colonoscopy. But, in order to be the most accurate in your screening, colonoscopy is the best. The good news is that if you do not have any risk factors, the colonoscopy is recommended every ten years; the recommendation is every year with risk factors. The risk factors for colorectal cancer are:

- You have had colorectal cancer before, even if it has been completely removed.
- You have a close relative (such as a sister, brother, parent, or child) who had colorectal polyps or colorectal cancer.
- You have a history of polyps.
- You have inflammatory bowel disease (like ulcerative colitis or Crohn's disease).

For men aged 50 years or better, prostate cancer screening is recommended. Prostate cancer is detected by measuring the prostate-specific antigen (PSA) level in the blood. Also, a rectal exam by a physician will show the size of the prostate and detect enlargement.

Prostate cancer has increased in the following groups:

- Those with a father, brother, or son who has had prostate cancer, especially if the relatives were young when they got the disease.

- African-Americans; prostate cancer is more common in this group for unknown reasons.

- Older men; approximately two out of every three prostate cancers are found in men over the age of 65.

Cerebrovascular Accident: This is commonly known as a stroke. There are some tests that may be able to assess if you are at risk for stroke, including carotid ultrasound, specialized MRIs, and angiography. These tests are only recommended for those with risk factors and are not for everyone.

The risk of stroke increases with age. Perhaps one of the most important ways to prevent the total incapacitation that may occur with stroke is to be able to recognize a stroke quickly. The best results occur when treatment is initiated within the first 60 minutes. Signs and symptoms of stroke are:

- Sudden numbness or weakness of the face, arm, or leg, especially on one side of the body

- Sudden confusion or trouble speaking or understanding speech

- Sudden trouble seeing in one or both eyes

- Sudden trouble walking, dizziness, or loss of balance or coordination

- Sudden severe headache with no known cause

These symptoms may occur for just several minutes and then go away. These are called "transient ischemic attacks" or "mini-strokes." These are your warning signs! If you have ever had any of these symptoms, they are a foreshadowing for the disaster that is building.

You are at risk for stroke if you have:

- High blood pressure that is uncontrolled
- Cigarette smoking habit
- Heart disease
- Diabetes
- Transient ischemic attacks (TIA) or previous stroke

Chronic Obstructive Pulmonary Disease (COPD): Nearly all cases of COPD can be prevented, because 80-90% are due to cigarette smoking. Never smoking or quitting smoking is the single most important step you can take to reduce your risk. There are other causes of COPD, which include exposure to environmental pollutants, repeated respiratory infections, and a genetic condition called Alpha-1-Antitrypsin Deficiency. Screening for those at risk of COPD include pulmonary function tests, chest X-ray, CT scan of the lungs, and blood tests for alpha-1-antitrypsin levels.

You are at increased risk for COPD if:

- You are a cigarette smoker.
- You have a genetic factor mentioned above.
- You are Caucasian.
- You are male, but this has been historically due to higher smoking rates in males; however, women are quickly catching up as the smoking rates continue to increase in women.
- You have exposure to environmental and occupational pollutants.
- You have frequent lung infections, especially as a child, as this can cause scarring in the lungs.

Pneumonia: Pneumonia affects people in all age groups, but the concern is that pneumonia can cause mortality in as many as 50% of seniors who are infected. Pneumonia most commonly is caused by bacteria, viruses, or mycoplasmas. Other causes include fungi, chemicals, aspirated food or liquid, and foreign objects. The single most preventive measure is hand washing and good hygiene. Smoking also increases the risk for pneumonia, as does living in a nursing home.

Vaccines available include the pneumococcal vaccine, which protects against a specific bacterial pneumonia, and the influenza vaccine, of which pneumonia may be a complication. Diet, regular exercise, and plenty of rest can help prevent pneumonia.

Those most at risk for pneumonia include:

- Age 65 or older
- Flu or other respiratory illness
- Chronic illness, such as heart disease or lung disease
- Stroke (aspiration pneumonia due to difficult swallowing)
- Weakened immune system caused by AIDS or chemotherapy treatment
- Chronic bronchitis
- Malnutrition
- Alcohol or drug abuse
- Smoking
- Chronic exposure to certain chemicals (for example, work in construction or agriculture)

Diabetes: According to the Centers for Disease Control and Prevention, between 1980 and 2004 the number of people with diabetes in the United States has doubled, and 40% of those with diabetes are over age 65. The total number of type 2 diabetics in 1994 was nearly 15 million.

The two most important ways to prevent diabetes are with weight loss and moderate exercise. These factors will guide you in knowing whether or not you are at risk for diabetes:

- I have a parent, brother, or sister with diabetes.

- My family background is Alaska Native, American Indian, African-American, Hispanic/Latino, Asian American, or Pacific Islander.

- I have had gestational diabetes, or I gave birth to at least one baby weighing more than nine pounds.

- My blood pressure is 140/90 mm Hg or higher, or I have been told that I have high blood pressure.

- My cholesterol levels are not normal; my HDL cholesterol ("good" cholesterol) is below 35 mg/dL, or my triglyceride level is above 250 mg/dL.

- I am fairly inactive; I exercise fewer than three times a week.

- I am a woman with polycystic ovary syndrome (also called PCOS).

- On previous testing, I had impaired glucose tolerance (IGT) or impaired fasting glucose (IFG).

- I have other clinical conditions associated with insulin resistance, such as acanthosis nigricans.

- I have a history of cardiovascular disease.

The more positive factors you have, the greater your risk for diabetes.

The glucose levels for the diagnosis of diabetes have become much more stringent over the last ten years. The current criteria are a random glucose (glucose that is taken at any time) greater than 200 mg/dL or a fasting glucose (fasting for at least eight hours) greater than 126 mg/dL.

Testing for diabetes is recommended starting at age 45 if there are no risk factors or symptoms. Symptoms include frequent urination, feeling thirsty, and unexplained weight loss. If normal, testing should be done at three-year intervals. If your Body Mass Index (BMI) is greater than 25 (see page 172), or if you have any of the risk factors above, the testing should be done more frequently.

For those who have the diagnosis of diabetes, lifestyle modification and medications are a must. The morbidity and mortality associated with diabetes are perhaps the most taxing on the health care system today. There is a direct correlation between diabetes and cardiovascular (heart) disease, nephropathy (kidney disease), retinopathy (disease of the retina in the eye,) and neuropathy (disease of the nerves). Tight control of blood glucose has proven to slow the diabetes disease process and its associated complications.

Accidents: Accidents are the seventh leading cause of death in people over age 65. Many times these are preventable, and being aware of the most common accidents in the home and outside of the home may be the best prevention.

Falls and resulting hip fractures are by far the most common disabling accidents in the elderly. Poor eyesight and hearing can decrease awareness of hazards. Arthritis, neurological disease, and impaired coordination and balance can make older adults unsteady as well.

Steps to take to decrease accidents in the home include:

- Light all stairways and have light switches at both the bottom and the top of the stairs.
- Use night lights or bedside remote-control light switches.
- Be sure both sides of stairways have sturdy handrails.

- Tack down carpeting on stairs and use nonskid treads.

- Remove throw rugs that tend to slide.

- Arrange furniture and other objects so they are not obstructing walkways.

- Use grab bars on bathroom walls and nonskid mats or strips in the bathtub.

- Keep outdoor steps and walkways in good repair.

Car accidents are the most common cause of accidental deaths among the 65-74-year-old age group. Your ability to drive safely may be affected by such age-related changes as sensitivity to glare, poor night vision, problems with coordination, and slower reaction times. You may want to make simple changes, such as driving only during the day, avoiding rush hour, driving less often and more slowly. Independence is always a difficult subject, but safety is always more important.

The best prevention for accidents is to be prepared. By identifying possible hazards and making good choices, most accidents can be avoided or the consequences can be diminished.

Septicemia: Septicemia is a bacterial infection in the blood. Most commonly in the elderly it stems from a urinary tract infection, but it can also come from pneumonia, bone infections, or meningitis. Septicemia can become very serious quickly and can cause death if not treated immediately. Most often, intravenous (IV) antibiotics are needed to treat this life-threatening condition. Prevention of septicemia includes treating infections promptly and receiving all of your proper vaccinations.

Nephritis: Nephritis is commonly known as kidney disease. Nephritis can be an acute or chronic condition. The main causes of chronic kidney disease are diabetes and high blood pressure. These are chronic conditions, and both uncontrolled diabetes and high blood pressure work on destroying the kidneys just a little bit at a time, day after day. This is why it is critical that chronic conditions are controlled. If not, they will eat away at the body.

You are at risk for kidney disease if you have the following risk factors:

- Diabetes
- Inflammation of the kidney
- High blood pressure
- Long-term infection
- Kidney stones causing urinary blockage
- Polycystic kidney disease, a genetic condition
- Certain medications; talk with your physician

Diagnosis of chronic kidney disease is done through blood testing and urine testing for protein. Symptoms may not be present until one-tenth of the kidney function is destroyed. The most important prevention is controlling blood sugar and high blood pressure. If you have any of these risk factors, you need to have a kidney check at least annually.

Alzheimer's Disease: Alzheimer's disease is perhaps the most debilitating and heart-wrenching chronic condition of the elderly today. Alzheimer's is a progressive disease in which the nerve cells in the brain slowly die, causing decreased mental function and, ultimately, death. The cause of Alzheimer's disease is unknown and there is no cure at this time, although if it is detected early, there are now medications that can slow the progression of the disease.

Because the cause of Alzheimer's disease is not yet clear, the only two risk factors are:

- Age
- Family history

Again, early diagnosis is the key. Therefore, family members and seniors both should know the warning signs of Alzheimer's disease:

- Memory loss
- Difficulty performing familiar tasks
- Problems with language
- Disorientation to time and place
- Poor or decreased judgment
- Problems with abstract thinking
- Misplacing things
- Changes in mood or behavior
- Changes in personality
- Loss of initiative

Most people associate the disease with not being able to remember. This is a key symptom, but forgetfulness may be a sign of routine aging. Knowing the other symptoms in combination with memory loss can lead to the proper diagnosis.

Immunizations: Shots are not just for kids any more. There are more and more vaccine recommendations every day. For the senior population, there are three main immunizations that are recommended for most people: influenza, pneumococcal, and hepatitis B.

- An influenza, or flu, shot is recommended for all people over age 65 every year. This annual vaccine protects against the respiratory illness. Unfortunately, the flu shot has a bad reputation, and there are a lot of misconceptions about what it protects against. Influenza, or the flu, is a viral respiratory illness spread by coughing or sneezing. Symptoms of the flu are fever, chills, headache, dry cough, runny or stuffy nose, sore throat, and muscle aches. The difference between influenza and the common cold is that the symptoms of influenza are more severe and the fatigue lasts much longer. The influenza vaccine does not protect against the "stomach flu," which is another set of viral illnesses.

There is also the misconception that you can get the flu from the flu shot. This is impossible due to the fact that the viruses in the shot are dead; therefore, they cannot cause disease.

If you do get the flu, see your doctor right away. There are medications that can help lessen both the symptoms and the duration.

- Pneumococcal vaccine is commonly known as the pneumonia shot. This vaccine is recommended for all healthy people age 65 and better. Younger populations may get the pneumonia shot if they have heart disease, lung disease, sickle cell disease, diabetes, alcoholism, cirrhosis of the liver, cancer, HIV, or a weakened immune system. These populations may need a second dose, especially if they are immunocompromised.

- Hepatitis B vaccine is recommended only in elderly populations with hemophilia, end stage kidney disease, or other diseases that weaken the immune system. There are other groups that should also get the hepatitis B vaccine if they have not. They include health care workers and those who may be exposed to people with hepatitis B.

Glaucoma: Glaucoma is the second leading cause of blindness in adults in the United States. There are two types of glaucoma — open angle and closed angle. Open angle glaucoma is the most common type and accounts for nearly 90% of cases. Open angle glaucoma is caused by increased fluid in the eye which pushes on the optic nerve, causing blindness. This fluid collection can occur very slowly, and symptoms may not show up until the late stages, when it may be too late. Closed angle glaucoma is also caused by a fluid build-up, but this tends to collect more quickly and cause severe eye pain.

As always, if you have risk factors, you should be screened more frequently and at an early age. The risk factors for developing glaucoma include:

- Being of African, Hispanic, Inuit, Irish, Japanese, Russian, or Scandinavian descent
- Family history of glaucoma
- Nearsightedness
- Age greater than 40
- Diabetes
- Previous eye trauma
- Steroid medication use

The good news about glaucoma is that if treated early, medications can be used to slow the progression of the disease and, hopefully, prevent blindness. The key to glaucoma is early detection and treatment.

Osteoporosis: Osteoporosis is a condition where the bones become thin and brittle and are more likely to break. Bone development occurs during childhood and adolescence. Without adequate calcium and vitamin D, the optimal bone density will not develop. This comes into play in the 30s when bones begin to degenerate. Bone loss tends to speed up in the 50s for women, when hormone levels decrease, and in the 60s for men.

Osteoporosis is a silent disease. You may never know that you have a problem until you have a broken hip or you suddenly lose one to two inches in height. At this point, it is too late to rebuild what you have lost.

Risk factors for osteoporosis include:

- Family history of osteoporosis
- Smoking
- Excessive alcohol use
- Sedentary lifestyle
- Hyperthyroidism or rheumatoid arthritis

Screening for osteoporosis should begin at age 65 for most women, age 60 for those with risk factors. A bone mineral density test is a mainstay for assessing bone density. Prevention, first and foremost, includes eating a balanced diet with calcium-rich foods, especially during childhood. Regular exercise and not smoking are crucial for bone health.

Enjoying the Golden Years

The decades of the 60s and beyond should be a time of relaxation and enjoyment. With proper care and "fine tuning" of your body, they can be filled with fun instead of physician visits and tests. Starting early with prevention and knowing your risk factors for chronic diseases can improve your quality of life, not just the quantity of life.

For more information, you can visit these Web sites: www.medicare.gov, www.webmd.com, and www.emedicine.com.

CHAPTER 4

Wellness and "Aunt Kit"

The responsibility of caring for senior citizens brings an entirely new challenge to the family unit today. What is the challenge? As was the custom and responsibility for our forefathers in their native countries, families in this country used to care for their senior loved ones until the Lord took them home. I recently asked a Vietnamese-born lady, who came to this country and became a citizen, what was the greatest difference she has observed between America and Vietnam. She quickly responded that there are no nursing homes in her home country.

You and I know that because of our family structure today, with both adults working and so many other family issues, many of our families' senior citizens become neglected or at least feel neglected. There is much that can and should be done.

As we think of our senior loved ones, we need to consider with them what the options are. In most cases there are two options for a senior loved one who has reached that point in life when he or she needs assistance in daily living. The first choice should always be to stay in the home of a child if at all possible.

I want to tell you the true story of an "at home" senior. It's a story that should make us all proud and remind us that the Lord always provides for His children when we put our faith and trust in Him.

This is a tribute to Louise "Aunt Kit" Hill, who lived in Bryant, Arkansas, a small, rural farming community. She and her husband

Ralph operated a dairy farm for many years. They raised four children, two sons, Herbert and Winfred, and two daughters, Marilyn and Colleen. They were lifelong Lutherans and supported their church in every way possible. When the Lord called Ralph home, Louise continued to be active and serve her church and her community. In fact, an entire book could be written about the Ralph and Louise Hill family and their contributions to church, community, and country.

When the time came that Aunt Kit needed assistance in her daily routine, her daughter Colleen and her husband made a decision that Aunt Kit would live with them. This meant Colleen became a full-time stay-at-home caregiver.

How did this affect family life? Aunt Kit's daughter, Colleen Hill Mays, has this to say about her mother's "Passion for Service":

> My mother, Anna Louise Hill, known commonly as Louise or Aunt Kit, died in her room in our home February 28, 2007. I always thought it would be an undesirable thing to have her die at home, but now I am very thankful for that event. Nearly every morning I go to her room, see the sun stream through the east window, and breathe the sweet fragrance of her lotion and powder that still lingers after her death. The hospital bed, the oxygen machine, the disposable diapers, the medicines, the toiletries, and all the other necessities for meeting her personal needs are all gone. My canopy bed, my baby dolls, her favorite pictures, and my favorite pictures of her and my daddy now fill the room.
>
> The things that are not visible to anyone, including me, are the memories from the many days and nights that she and I shared the room for the past five years. There was never a decision to be made about whether Mother would live with my husband Doug and me or whether she would live out her life in a facility for the elderly. One reason was because Mother never was elderly, even though she died at the age of 98 years, 6 months, and 12 days.

I cannot remember a time that Mother did not work hard. Maybe that's one of the reasons for her longevity. Mother and Daddy married in 1929 and not long after began dairy farming in Bryant, Arkansas. During those tough years in world history, Mother worked at milking, farming, raising a garden, and then raising a family. As the years went by, many nieces, nephews, and local townspeople worked on the dairy farm. My husband, Doug, thinks it was sort of like a penal farm, but I think it was rather an opportunity for employment.

As years went by, Mother became the cook, housekeeper, laundress, and mother to all of these people because they not only worked on the farm, they lived and ate in the home with Mother and Daddy. One of my cousins remembers he was just a young teenager when he worked there and could hardly wait to be called to lunch, because he was always so excited about the wonderful meal Mother would have fixed. I have often wondered how she had things to cook and prepare, because there were no Wal-Mart Supercenters back in the 1930s and 1940s. Somehow she prepared memorable, nourishing meals for the family and the hired help.

Mother was sick a lot when I was a kid, so I spent a lot of time with my Aunt Florence and Uncle Ed Parker. I wonder where the other kids went? I guess they were old enough to take care of themselves! My sister, Marilyn, and my brothers, Herbie and Wimp, were older than me. By the time I was nine years old, Mother began being healthy and was never sick or ailing in any way I can remember until 1998. That year, she began having some congestive heart failure problems. It was a year before I was planning to retire from my public school teaching career. I missed many days that year until her health stabilized. The following year proved to be an even worse year for Mother, so I retired from teaching after 29 years of service.

I retired in 2000, and believe it or not, Mother got better. I had completed a career of working with teenagers, and I knew and had made it known that my next career would be caring for the elderly. I didn't know I would get a full-time job so quickly. Doug has reminded me many times in the last few years to be careful what you wish for, because sometimes you get those very things. I know now that God was giving me time to rest and get caught up with things in my life in preparation for caring for Mother in the years to come.

She came to live with us in April 2002. We went through lots of hospital stays in the next couple of years, but with the help of God and a wonderful doctor, and monitoring her condition and her medication on a daily basis, we were able to stay out of the hospital so often. I cannot tell you that all days were wonderful and great. The phrase Doug uses: you turn in your "fun card."

Caring for the elderly is like caring for a baby, but your baby is getting weaker and becoming more dependent; whereas an infant is getting stronger and becoming independent. Some days the care is very demanding and very confining. You must have sitters to be able to leave home, you sleep with a baby monitor next to your ear, and you spend some days and nights next to the bed without leaving. You depend on family and friends to relieve you, and it's not always easy to ask for nor accept that help.

As Mother began to weaken, I was encouraged to engage the local hospice organization to help. We had wonderful hospice people for the last two years of Mother's life. Our two favorite care givers, Fran and Tina, were here all day the day Mother died. That evening when she died, they bathed her, prepared her body, and dressed her body in a pretty pink robe with little rosebuds that matched her new blankets for her trip to the mortuary. They were a true blessing to Mother and me.

Mother was always a very active person in many organizations. I remember when I was a kid, she was a member of the Bryant Study Club. I could never understand what they studied, but I think it must have been sort of like Oprah's

Book Club. I think people read and reported on books and then discussed them. Who knows?

Mother loved to host things like that and the Home Demonstration Club, and of course, the Ladies Aid from Immanuel Lutheran Church at Alexander. She was quite the hostess and quite the cook. On one occasion when the Study Club was meeting at our house with all of the town's "little ladies" present, Daddy paraded through their midst dressed in his underwear and Mother's three-quarter length coat. What a frightening sight! What skinny, naked, bird legs he displayed from under that pretty gray coat. Mother and those little ladies never got over that evening. He was having fun, but she was so embarrassed.

When I reached school age, Mother went to work outside the home. She was a teacher's assistant to Edith Reinke at First Lutheran School in Little Rock. Can you imagine there being teacher's assistants in 1951? People today think that is a new position in schools. She worked in the cafeteria there also. She went on to do many public work jobs after that. The dairy business had grown and had hired hands to do a lot of the work, and of course, there were growing kids to work then too. She worked at a retail store, a retail bakery, a department store, and ended her paid working career as a civilian employee of the U.S. Postal Service in Bryant.

It goes without saying that Mother was a woman of faith. She was always active in the Lutheran Church. She taught Sunday School for many years and was an active member of the Lutheran Women's Missionary League, the Ladies Aid at Immanuel, and the Evening Guild at First Lutheran in Benton. She sang in the choirs of the two churches and was active in every part of church life. Late in life, she became a volunteer at Saline Memorial Hospital in Benton. She volunteered 5,500 hours, stopping at the age of 92 when her health began to fail.

I can remember Mother always being busy with her

hands. As a young girl, she made the dresses and clothes for herself and her sisters. Her mother died when she was 14 or 15 years old, so she had to grow up fast. She was always piecing quilts, quilting, making clothes for us kids and herself. Embroidering, crocheting, you name it, she did it.

I was in the ninth grade when she worked at the bakery. She got the owners to let her bring her sewing machine to work, where she made clothes for us and Barbie doll clothes between customers. What employers would allow that today?

In the late 1970s Mother crocheted dolls that were made together with their blanket. When she would finish each one, she would wrap up the "baby" in the blanket, then rock it in her arms and sing and talk to it. Daddy thought she was "off her rocker." She made dozens of those dolls in all colors and sold them along with her embroidered, hand-quilted quilts. There are still a lot of those items in the community today.

I never knew why my sister and I had so many dolls when we were kids, but I found out at the Ladies Candlelight Dinner at Zion Lutheran Church in December of 2004. Mother was asked to speak and tell about her Christmases as a child. That night she gave us quite a Christmas story. I found out then that one of her greatest loves was the love of dolls. That helped me understand a lot about things she had done, like getting my old dolls out of the attic, making new clothes for them, and giving them back to me after I was an adult. They are now residents in "her room" in our home. What treasures!

Mother cared for my daddy when he was homebound and finally bedfast. I never appreciated what my mother did for Daddy until I got to do the same care giving for her. There was a big difference, however – Mother was 86 when Daddy died, and I am 62. I don't know how she was able to care for him and continue to do all the other things she did. Her method of coping with the day-to-day challenges was working with her sewing and service projects. My method of coping was working outdoors and spending time with our donkeys, goats, dog, and cats. They are always thrilled to see me; they love unconditionally.

Mother never lost her desire to sew and serve. She began a sewing group in her home in 1984. Most of the women were from Immanuel Lutheran in Alexander. The group later moved to the church to meet as a group to do service projects. They took donated fabric scraps or yardage, used templates to mark blocks, and cut the blocks of fabric to make quilts for Lutheran World Relief.

Mother's favorite part was sewing the blocks together to form the quilt tops. They also made lap covers from blocks and gave them to hospitals, homes for unwed mothers, hospice programs, and nursing homes – anywhere there was a need.

She was passionate about this service. That group, made up of eight or ten aging ladies and a couple of young ones, could dream up more things to do with fabric than one can imagine. I never could understand cutting fabric apart to make blocks to sew back together! Just didn't make sense to me. Why not leave it in big pieces?

Ladies of the group began to age and fail in health, then they began to go to heaven. The group was dwindling, but Mother's passion never faltered. She nearly drove poor Mary Winkler nuts trying to get her to get that group going again. Keep in mind Mother was homebound but still "in charge." Mary's husband was very sick in the hospital for several months, and the Lord called him home in April 2006. Mary was weary, but Mother seemed rested. She continued to want things done.

One of the greatest benefits and blessings of keeping Mother in our home was that she was able to maintain the same quality of life to which she was accustomed. That included her being able to do her "thing." She had a very strict routine. She came to the kitchen on her walker around 7 a.m. for her breakfast. She went back to her room, read her devotion, and sewed or cut blocks until 9 a.m. Then it was time for "Good Morning Arkansas," when she got back in her hospital bed and crocheted on her baby caps for Children's Hospital until 10 a.m. Everything stopped at 10 a.m. for "The Price Is Right!"

At 11 a.m. there was a soap opera. At 12 noon there was lunch in the kitchen, then back to the room to cut blocks or crochet or nap until 3 p.m., when a game show came on. Oh, she was often frustrated if a visitor came or if hospice came for her bath during one of those "important shows." She watched a lot of televised golf and baseball on Saturday, but never did a single chore on Sunday. She said, "You are not supposed to work on Sunday," so she didn't. She watched two or three church services on Sunday morning television.

I cannot tell you that all day, every day was wonderful and easy. Mother and I were both control freaks with very strong wills, so you can imagine that we had some difficult decision making times. She usually won, with me feeling guilty and frustrated. Most of our problems were over the right pattern of blocks arranged together or getting more fabric from the sewing room at church "right now" so she didn't miss a lick.

I was blessed with many friends and relatives who would sit with Mother so I could do chores, doctor's appointments, shopping, etc. Jeanette Maertens Irby has been my best friend forever, and she could and would make Mother so happy because she would cut those blocks with her and arrange them in "just the perfect way." Mother looked forward to her coming, because Jeanette always humored her and let her have her way.

Mother's mind was perfect, but her body was failing. She could only continue her work through those of us who enabled her by doing some of the work for her.

In 2005 and 2006 she pieced 119 quilt tops and, I think, 76 lap covers. In 2006 she embroidered 11 pairs of pillowcases to give as Christmas gifts to her care givers and friends. That same year she crocheted 84 caps for the Children's Hospital. She kept trying and trying to get someone to complete the quilts and lap covers. I made a few suggestions, but my suggestions were always turned down. Finally, in February 2007 she joined the Lutheran Women's Missionary League at Zion Lutheran Church, where I am a member. That group took on the project of completing the quilts and lap covers that the Immanuel group had left unfinished and the ones she had made while she was homebound. Mother never got to attend a meeting nor a work day when they worked on the quilt tops.

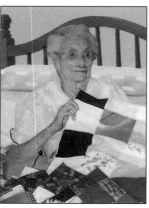

Aunt Kit

After Bible Study in our home on January 11, 2007, Mother fell when she got up to take off her robe. Nothing was broken, but she was cut and bruised from the fall. She was completely bedfast after that.

We went through three or four weeks when she was very miserable with pain and probably some depression, because it was becoming obvious that she was weakening. She had been on a morphine patch for four years because of compression fractures in her back, but now the dosage had to be increased, and she just could not get the strength to crochet any more. I felt like her days of service were over. Little did I know!

The week before she died, Mother could not get comfortable with her bed covers. They were too big, too heavy, too hot, not warm enough, wrong color — whatever! One day I got out a bolt of flannel that she had used to make baby blankets for the layette kits for World Relief, and I made two blankets. The fabric was pink with little rosebuds all over.

I made a blanket to fit her hospital bed from one thickness, and I made a second blanket of two thicknesses. When I took them to her room, she was thrilled; now she had one, two, or three thicknesses, they fit her bed, and she could regulate the temperature to her liking. What that also did was stimulate her service mind. She said, "Friends in Christ Lutheran at Bryant need baby blankets for their Baskets of Hope. I think I can make some for them from this fabric. Is there any left?"

I said, "Mother you can't even sit up, how can you sew?" She said, "I don't know, but I can try to sit at the machine for a few minutes at a time."

Her passion was still there! I started cutting and washing fabric and made plans to rearrange the room once more to open the sewing machine.

The Lord had other plans for Mother. He took her to Himself about a week later. She died on the same date on which my friend Jeanette's mother had died in 1998. Jeanette's mother and my mother were best friends when they were kids and teenagers, and now, 80 plus years later we are best friends. Mother and Clara Maertens were buried on the same date, and the same songs were used for their funeral services – without us knowing it until the service plans were complete. If anyone doubts the power and might of our Lord, sit with me for a while and I can tell you unbelievable things that have happened for and to me in the past four months.

About a month before Mother's death, I reached a real "valley" of my life. I had had amazing support and love from my family, my husband, my friends, and my Bible classes, but my very nature of control had become a stumbling block. I had tried to control many things in my life, including the time and method and circumstances of my mother's death.

At the point of physical, emotional, and mental break-down, I finally let go and let God. He lifted my burden, and miraculous things began to happen in her life and mine. He took her home, and He gave me such peace in her leaving me. I will forever miss her in our home and my life, but as I told her at the moment of her death, I will see her again in just a little while. I can't wait to tell her that the Zion sewing group finished 17 of the quilts on the first day they met. They will all be finished soon.

The day before Mother died, my second mother, Aunt Florence, fell and broke a hip. She had cared for 45 foster children during her adult years and still was keeping one of them in her home when she fell. One of those foster children, Cindy Miller, is 47 years old and was dependent on her "mother" for 41 years. The day Mother died, Aunt Florence had surgery and I had to find a state facility for Cindy.

This is a whole different story, but it all points to God's control and work in my life. He provided a place for Cindy the day I needed it – virtually impossible in my eyes.

Two days after Mother's burial I had to make the decision to place Aunt Florence in a nursing/rehabilitation facility – virtually impossible in my eyes to find a place near me, but you know God.

On March 13, Aunt Florence's 98th birthday, God called her home. In a week and a half God had taken care of my every need with the elderly and handicapped loved ones who depended on me.

I pray He will now give me the strength, courage, and patience to live without my mothers. I have relationship rebuilding to do with my husband, who has been so patient and helpful to me. He has been sort of "put on the back burner" for several years. He, too, loved and cared for Mother and Daddy. I will continue to monitor Cindy's care in her new home. When I rest up some, I plan to help other care givers as my friends have helped me.

Mother has been gone almost two months, and only yesterday did I realize that her real passion to serve began when she was about 75 years old. I am only 62. What does

God have in mind for me? How will He use me? I hope He doesn't need me to make quilts! Surely I have some other gifts.

Mother and I had lots of time to talk in the last five years. Boy did we have some talks, and I got to do some preaching, too. She even talked a lot during the night when she did not know she was talking, but I sure was listening. She gave me specific details one night in her sleep of how to plant potatoes in a bushel basket. She talked a lot to and about the ones who had gone on before, and I know that she is telling them now lots of things that happened in her 98 plus years. What a great reunion it will be when we all get to Heaven!

God grant me the desire, passion, and strength that my mother had to serve Him and others.

I know He commanded us to honor our father and mother. It was such an honor for me to care for Mother. I know I served Him and honored my father and my mother by caring for her. Thank you, Lord, for that opportunity. ～

And what about Aunt Kit, with her ups and downs, taking life one day at a time at 98 years of age? She still had her daily routine. She made quilts and other items for Lutheran World Relief. Aunt Kit was happy and lived a full and productive life.

This is how the Lord intended the family to function. The family and the church have a real responsibility to our senior citizens. Colleen and her family are and will continue to be blessed for making this kind of wellness commitment to their loved one.

Aunt Kit's nephew, Johnny Farchman, had this to say about Aunt Kit and her family:

Anna Louise (Aunt Kit) Farchman Hill, a dedicated Christian, wife, mother, grandmother, great-grandmother, great-great-grandmother, daughter, sister, and aunt. Dedicated to her Lord and family for so very many years. When her father, John W. Farchman, in his later years needed some place to live, she and Uncle Ralph took him in, where he lived until his death in 1953. He, being an immigrant from Germany in the 1950s, not able to speak English upon arrival, would not allow German to be spoken in the Farchman household; the children received much harassment in school during World War I, so that my grandfather changed the spelling of the family name from "Farchmin" to "Farchman." This is something Aunt Kit would remember. Aunt Kit Hill will always, in my mind, fit the category of a "good and faithful" Christian.

John H. (Johnny) Farchman

Quilt of Holes

As I faced my Maker at the last judgment, I knelt before the Lord along with all the other souls. Before each of us laid our lives like the squares of a quilt in many piles. An angel sat before each of us, sewing our quilt squares together into a tapestry that is our life.

As my angel took each piece of cloth off the pile, I noticed how ragged and empty each of my squares was. They were filled with giant holes. Each square was labeled with a part of my life that had been difficult, the challenges and temptations I was faced with in everyday life. I saw hardships that I endured, which were the largest holes of all.

I glanced around me. Nobody else had such squares. Other than a tiny hole here and there, the other tapestries were filled with rich color and the bright hues of worldly fortune.

I gazed upon my own life and was disheartened. My angel was sewing the ragged pieces of cloth together, threadbare and empty, like binding air.

Finally, the time came when each life was to be displayed, held up to the light and the scrutiny of truth. The others rose; each in turn, holding up their tapestries. So filled their lives had been.

My angel looked at me and nodded for me to rise. My gaze dropped to the ground in shame. I hadn't had all the earthly fortunes. I had love in my life and laughter, but there had also been trials of illness and wealth and false accusations that took from me my world as I knew it.

I had to start over many times. I often struggled with the temptation to quit, only to somehow muster the strength to pick up and begin again. I spent many nights on my knees in prayer, asking for help and guidance in my life. I had often been held up to ridicule, which I endured painfully, each time offering it up to the Father in hopes that I would not melt within my skin beneath the judgmental gaze of those who unfairly judged me.

Now, I had to face the truth. My life was what it was, and I had to accept it for what it was. I rose and slowly lifted the combined squares of my life to the light.

An awe-filled gasp filled the air. I gazed around at the others who stared at me with wide eyes. Then, I looked upon the tapestry before me. Light flooded the many holes creating an image, the face of Christ. Then our Lord stood before me with warmth and love in His eyes. He said, "Every time you gave over your life to Me, it became My life, My hardships, and My struggles. Each point of light in your life is when you stepped aside and let Me shine through, until there was more of Me than there was of you."

May all our quilts be threadbare and worn, allowing Christ to shine through!

Author Unknown

CHAPTER 5

Wellness Ministry and Your Congregation

Let me tell you about a commercial I heard recently. It goes like this:

> Mrs. Riley lives on the second floor. She looks out her window and listens to the neighbors as they walk by. She almost got a hot meal, but then Mrs. Richy walked on by. She almost went to the doctor today, but then Mrs. Rice forgot to stop by. She almost got the latest news from church, but Pastor did not make it by. Maybe tomorrow, will you stop by?

Congregations and groups within the church, such as the Ladies Aid, men's organizations, and others, should have a wellness program that includes ministry to seniors. Zion Lutheran Church in Corunna, Indiana, almost by accident, started a spiritual wellness program that still flourishes today.

The program for senior citizens started when Elders Donald Martz and David Swogger and a pastor were trying to locate a senior citizen. A congregant on the church's membership list, the gentleman had moved three times. They finally found him in a nursing home about 53 miles from the church.

After a visit, Donald, David, and the pastor asked the nursing home social worker if they could arrange for the chaplain or pastor to minister to our member. Let them tell the story from here:

> The social worker told us there was no minister who served the home on a regular basis. We talked and decided that

maybe the Lord was challenging us to minister to the people in this nursing home.

A decision was made that Zion would serve this nursing facility. Plans were made for our congregation to visit the home every Saturday at 10:30 a.m.

The first Saturday we met in the dining area where we sang some songs and had a devotion with about ten residents from this meager beginning and travel of 53 miles one way. Each time we left we would ask each other if it were really worth it, and each time we would agree that it was worth it.

Six years later, Zion Lutheran Church continues to serve the first venture and by the grace of God we now serve four other facilities with Bible Class and church services.

What about the possibilities in your congregation? Talk with your pastor and see what you can do. If you have a parish nurse, work with her in setting up a wellness program. Congregations and their leaders have a real opportunity to initiate programs in wellness that reach out to the community as well as serve their own members.

A health care physician recently pointed out that we all know very well the importance of wellness and a healthy lifestyle for our church workers and individual family members. We know that living a healthy life is important at every age.

We are told that obesity is a national epidemic at all levels in our society. For the first time in a decade, life expectancy has declined rather than increased, and the culprit is unhealthy lifestyles.

The federal government has finalized rules that govern the way companies can encourage employees to develop healthier lifestyles. Why? Because it is widely recognized that there is a serious health problem in America. The question is: Where does wellness and a healthy lifestyle rank with us, our families, and our church and its workers? Most congregations have no plan or valuable tools other than those congregations that are fortunate enough to have a parish nurse. These angels of health and wellness are doing an outstanding job. Unfortunately, they have limited resources and most are volunteers. They need more resources and tools to work within their congregations.

As a synod, our districts and local congregations need to identify the issues in our lifestyles that are causing the challenge and then address these issues. There are two areas of wellness challenge. The first is spiritual health. Spiritual health means what my relationship with God is as I relate to Him through Jesus Christ my Savior by the power of the Holy Spirit, working first through baptism, water and the Word, then through the Word and Holy Communion.

Through our baptism we were brought back into a proper relationship with God our Heavenly Father. What benefit does baptism give to the person receiving it? It works forgiveness of sins, rescues from death and the devil, and gives eternal salvation to all who believe this as the words and promises of God declare according to Luther's Small Catechism.

And what about the Lord's Supper? Luther tells us what the benefits are of this drinking with these words: "Given and shed for you for the forgiveness of sins."

The Bible shows us that in the Sacrament there is forgiveness of sins, life, and salvation. Where there is forgiveness of sins, there is also life and salvation. A professor once told me that people could be around the Word all their lives and still be lost. I was startled at the time, but the point he was making is that we can become so busy with important and good things that we neglect the one thing needful. Remember Martha in Luke 10:40: "'Martha, Martha', the Lord answered, 'you are worried and upset about many things but only one thing is needed.'"

The point is that God wants His children — pastors, teachers, moms, dads, children, aunts — to use their time as children of the Heavenly Father. I recently asked a wellness class that I was teaching to outline a spiritual wellness plan. Every student's concern is enough time during the day. If we are not spiritually fed in the proper way, it affects the body as an individual and each family member in some way. Are we so busy that we do not have time for family devotions, Sunday School, adult Bible Class, and worship?

A pastor tells this account of his lifestyle:

> I thought I had to do everything, lead all of the meetings in our church, teach all of the classes, etc. I was afraid to delegate any responsibilities. My elders were wallflowers, and the church council I expected to rubber stamp. I had little or no time for hospital calls and home visits. The rest of the time was on the computer. My family missed me, and my church missed me. I thought I was the only one who could do our ministry in the proper way.

This pastor said it took him and his elders a year to get him and the congregation really functioning in Word and Sacrament ministry.

Congregations may want to assess ministry in the congregation by asking and addressing these questions:

1. Is every member in adult Bible Class? If not, why not and what do we need to do to get them in Bible study?

2. What are we doing about our numbers who attend church and the Lord's Supper infrequently? What do we mean by infrequently?

3. Is there a scope and sequence in our Sunday School curriculum, and does the pastor go over the lessons with our teachers every month?

4. How does each group in our church tie into Word and Sacrament ministry?

5. Is our Youth Group a part of Word and Sacrament ministry?

6. Are our seniors a part of Word and Sacrament ministry? Nursing home ministry? Home care ministry?

7. Do we have a wellness committee and how does it function?

8. If we have an elementary school and/or high school, how does the school fit into Word and Sacrament ministry?

9. Have we as a congregation identified what Word and Sacrament mean to us?

Wellness involves my whole life in Christ, and who I am in Him determines how I will live in relation to others. We serve God and our neighbor. My body is a temple of the Holy Spirit, a vessel or tool which God uses so that I might serve Him. The choices I make with my body, mind, and lifestyle may positively or negatively affect my ability to serve Him. Lifestyle choices begin at birth and stay with us until death.

It is a proven fact that when we make the proper lifestyle choices, our quality of life, our quality of health, and our longevity of life are extended. Our desire, then, is to help our people make the proper lifestyle choices.

To help our people in the congregation, Concordia Plan Services offers this suggested composition for a church wellness committee:

1. A senior citizen, age 65 or older

2. A middle-aged adult, age 30-50

3. A high school senior or college student

4. A single adult

The recommendation continues, outlining these actions and functions for the wellness committee:

A. Elect a chairperson and secretary.

B. The chairperson should serve on the Church Council and give reports to the Council on activities concerning wellness in the congregation.

C. Work with the parish nurse and help implement recommended programs and activities.

D. Work with congregation leaders and members to develop realistic wellness activities that lead to awareness and healthy lifestyles for workers and members.

E. Host seminars on wellness and promote health risk assessments.

F. Coordinate with Concordia Plan Services and become familiar with the "Be Well-Serve Well" program benefits which include a health risk assessment, health advisor program, 24-hour nurse line, disease management, lifestyle management, and Web-based online tools.

G. Know the six areas that individuals can control and the steps necessary to get them under control:

1. Blood pressure: It can be controlled and it must be controlled. Ideal blood pressure should be below 120/80.

2. Cholesterol: It too can be controlled and must be controlled. Ideal cholesterol counts are:

   Total: Below 200 mg/dL

   LDL: Below 100 mg/dL

   HDL: Above 40

3. Smoking: No excuse, no exception. Stop now.

4. Diet: Manage portion control.

5. Exercise: The American Heart Association recommends exercise one hour per day, seven days a week.

6. Body Mass Index: Body mass index (BMI) is the ratio of weight to height. The higher your BMI, the greater the risk of high blood pressure and diabetes. A normal BMI is 18.5-24; ask your doctor to determine your BMI or refer to the National Heart Lung Blood Institute chart on page 172.

These six areas are excellent ways to take care of the temple which is your body.

I would like to bring a team to your church, school, or community to conduct a complete wellness seminar and help you know more. We can train people, in addition to your parish nurse, to implement an ongoing wellness program in your area. We can also demonstrate an exercise program you can use at home or wherever you are with little or no equipment. We begin slowly and work up to one hour per day, four days a week.

For a set of wellness materials that are available through CTS Family Press, please e-mail or write to me:

Rev. Al Wingfield
CTS Family Press
6600 North Clinton Street
Fort Wayne, Indiana 46825

Telephone: (260) 452-2106

Fax: (260) 452-2121

E-mail: al@alwingfield.com

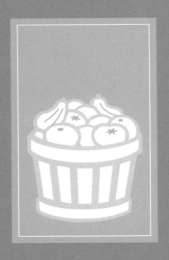

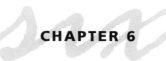

CHAPTER 6

Wellness Eating

As the saying goes, "we are what we eat." Food and portion control is absolutely necessary for your wellness plan. The information in this chapter will help you plan menus for you and your family to be able to eat healthy and to control your portions.

In addition to the healthy eating information provided here, you may want to visit the United States Department of Agriculture's (USDA) Web site, www.mypyramid.gov, which offers a wealth of detailed information. Designed to help Americans live longer, better and healthier lives, the "MyPyramid" replaces the Food Guide Pyramid introduced in 1992. It is one part of the USDA's overall food guidance system that emphasizes the need for a more individualized approach to improving diet and lifestyle.

Combined with exercise, diet will help us "to be well, to serve well."

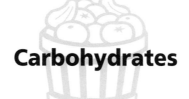

Carbohydrates

Carbohydrates (carbs) are composed of oxygen, carbon, and hydrogen. They are the basic fuel source for the body. Sugars, starches, and cellulose are the main forms in which carbohydrates occur in food. Starches and sugars are the major source of energy and the cheapest and most easily used form of fuel for the body. When digested, carbs are changed to glycose and glucose; when they are broken down into the sugars, they are used for energy-fuel. Some excess can be stored for future use as energy-fuel, but this amount is limited. The rest is stored as body fat. Carbohydrates also encourage the growth of beneficial bacteria in the intestines and also aid in the absorption of calcium and phosphorus.

Rice, pasta, bread, legumes, potatoes, starchy vegetables (corn, peas, and some beans) are the most commonly seen carbs in our diets. Fruits are a less concentrated source of carbohydrates because of their high water content. Watermelon and cantaloupe are the lowest in carb content, while bananas are among the highest. Dried fruits are higher in sugars because of the low moisture content. Carbohydrates are burned quickly and are either used for immediate fuel or, in the case of excess carb consumption, are converted to sugars and stored as fat.

Sugars

Sugar	Fructose	Corn Syrup
Sucrose	Maltose	High-Fructose
Glucose	Lactose	Corn Syrup
Dextrose	Mannitol	Molasses
Sorbitol	Honey	Maple Syrup

Food labeling is listed in the order of the weight of the ingredient items. Any or many of these items listed in the first few ingredients will likely be "empty calories."

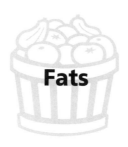

Fats

Lipid is the scientific name for fat. It applies to a group of substances, both animal and plant, that have a greasy, oily, or waxy consistency. All lipids are insoluble in water and contain one or more fatty acids in their chemical structure. There are more than 29 different fatty acids. All fats and oils, regardless of their fatty acid content, have the same energy value.

Before food fats can be absorbed into the bloodstream, they must be reduced to simpler compounds. Only about 1/3 of the fat in the intestine is completely broken down to fatty acids and glycerol; the remainder is absorbed in a partially digested state. Normally 95% or more of dietary fat is absorbed.

Some facts about fats:

- Essential fatty acids are necessary for the normal function of all tissue, however, in small amounts. Fats serve as carriers of fat-soluble vitamins A, D, E, and K.

- Fats are a reserve form of energy when food intake is low or when illness is present.

- Fat helps to maintain body temperature.

- Fat helps to protect internal organs by holding them in position and cushioning them from trauma. Too much fat will crowd organs, however.

- Fat prolongs the feeling of fullness and delays the onset of hunger pains.

- Shellfish are practically fat-free, while mackerel, tuna, salmon, and herring are fatty fish. However, they are still lower than most cuts of red meat.

- Red meat with marbled fat contains more saturated fat, because it cannot be trimmed away.

- Luncheon meats are high in fat.

- Vegetable oil is 100% fat.

- Other sources of plant fat come from nuts, seeds, coconut, olives, avocados, and palm oil.

- Baked products have hidden fats, because we do not see the egg yolks, butter, oils, etc.

- What is the difference in saturated and unsaturated fats?

  Saturated fatty acids are usually found in animal sources and are said to have an elevating effect on blood cholesterol. A fat is determined to be saturated if many hydrogen atoms are attached to the carbon atoms.

  Unsaturated fatty acids are mainly from plant/vegetable sources.

Heartful Health
Learning About Lipids

Item	Goal Range	Affected By
Total Cholesterol	below 200 mg/dL	diet, genetics
HDL (good cholesterol)	Women: above 50 mg/dL Men: above 40 mg/dL	smoking, exercise
LDL (bad cholesterol)	below 100 mg/dL (esablished heart disease) below 130 mg/dL (preventive)	diet (saturated fat)
Cholesterol/HDL ratio	Women: below 4.0 mg/dL Men: below 4.5 mg/dL	
Triglycerides	below 150 mg/dL	excess calories (fat, sugar, alcohol)
Glucose	70-110 mg/dL	

Good Fat List
1-3 servings per day of these good types of fat

Margarine (liquid oil should be the first ingredient)...................1 tsp.
    (Shedd's Spread®, Fleischmann's®, Mazola®, Chiffon®, Promise®,
    Olivio®, Parkay Gold®)

Diet Margarine..1 Tbsp.

Fat-free Spreads..Free

Oil (preferably olive or canola)...1 tsp.

Nonstick cooking spray (e.g., PAM®)..Free

Salad dressings like French, Italian, Western, etc..................1 Tbsp.

Reduced-calorie salad dressings...2 Tbsp.

Fat-free salad dressings..Free

Mayonnaise..1 tsp.

Reduced-calorie mayonnaise..1 Tbsp.

Fat-free mayonnaise...Free

Fat-free cream cheese...1 Tbsp.

Fat-free sour cream...1 Tbsp., Free

Miracle Whip®...2 tsp.

Fat-free Miracle Whip®...Free

Avocado...1/8

Natural peanut butter (e.g., Smuckers®)..................................2 tsp.
    (Avoid regular peanut butter like Peter Pan® or Jif®;
    they contain hydrogenated fats)

Olives...10 small or 5 large

Nuts/Seeds (if salted)...1 Tbsp. (approx.)

Peanuts (1/2 ounce) (if salted)..........................20 small or 10 large

Doritos® Light tortilla chips..1 oz.

Regular tortilla chips...1/2 oz.

Taco shell...1 oz.

Many products, such as those below, can be made at home with or without fats. If you use fat, you must count these in your daily allowance of fat, and you should use canola oil. Also, try reducing the fat by substituting applesauce, juice, milk, or water for part of the fat.

Cake, unfrosted..2" square

Cupcake...1 average

Cookies..2 average

Banana Bread...1/16 loaf

Biscuit..1-2" diameter

Corn Bread...2" square

Muffin...1 average

Pancakes...2, 4" each

Waffles...1/4 of 9" round

Avoid Saturated Fats

Butter	Cream
Cream Cheese	Chocolate
Coconut	Palm Oil
Lard	Bacon Fat
Shortening	Meat Drippings
Coconut Oil	Stick Margarine

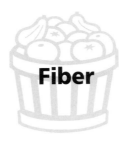

Fiber

What is fiber? It is a group of compounds found in plant foods. These compounds cannot be broken down by acids or enzymes in the digestive tract and are, therefore, eliminated through the bowel.

Soluble fiber (pectins, gums, guar, hemicellulose, oats, barley, some vegetables, and fruit)

- Delays gastric emptying time.
- Prolongs intestinal transit time.
- Flattens blood sugar rise after meals.
- Reduces serum cholesterol.

Insoluble fiber (cellulose, lignin, whole grain wheat, vegetables, fruit, corn bran, and nuts)

- Speeds gastric emptying time.
- Speeds intestinal transit.
- Has little effect on after meal sugar rise.
- Has minimal effect on serum cholesterol.

How Does Fiber Promote Good Health?

Fiber decreases constipation and reduces pressure in the intestinal tract, therefore, lowering the likelihood of diverticulosis, appendicitis, and hemorrhoids. The risk for colon cancer can be lowered with a fiber rich diet because the cancer causing agents can be diluted by fiber and moved more swiftly out of the intestinal tract.

Note that high fiber foods may interfere with the absorption of some minerals, including zinc, calcium, iron, and magnesium.

Supplements should be taken one hour prior or one hour after high fiber meals.

Increasing fiber intake should be done slowly. If increased too rapidly, cramping, gaseousness, and even diarrhea may occur. These symptoms are generally temporary. When increasing fiber intake, always increase water consumption. Without additional water, the gel-like fiber substance is not easily moved in the intestinal tract.

Fruits
Include 4-5 servings per day

Include

Apples, applesauce, apricots, bananas, blackberries, blueberries, cantaloupe, cherries, dates, dried apricots, figs, fruit cocktail, grapefruit, grapes, honeydew melon, kiwi, mandarin oranges, mangos, nectarines, oranges, papaya, peaches, pears, persimmons, pineapple, plums, pomegranates, prunes, raisins, raspberries, strawberries, tangerines, watermelon, and all fruit juices

Avoid

None

Grains
Include 6-8 servings per day

Include

Most yeast breads (whole grains are best), bagels, English muffins, whole wheat breads, French bread, pita bread, rye bread, pretzels, hard rolls, breadsticks (unbuttered), pizza crust (not pan fried), sandwich and hamburger buns

Most cereals (whole grains are best), oatmeal, bran flakes, Total®, Raisin Bran®, Quaker Oat Bran®, Shredded Wheat®, Fiber One®, Bran Buds®, Fruit 'n Fiber®, Meuslix®, Grape-Nuts®, Cheerios®, Kenmei Rice Bran®, Wheat Chex®, Wheaties®, Just Right ®

Crackers (3 gm. fat or less per ounce), saltines, Rye or Wheat Krisp®, Harvest Krisp®, Wasa®, Finn Crisp®, oyster, Sea Rounds®, Stoned Wheat Thins®, Triscuits®, Uneeda®, graham, zweiback toast, Pepperidge Farms English Water Biscuit®, Nabisco®, Crown Pilot®, Estee Wheat Wafers®, Health Valley Crackers®, Whole Wheat Premiums®

Other grain products:
Rice (brown rice is best)
Pasta (spaghetti, macaroni, etc.)
Tortillas (flour or corn)

Avoid

Doughnuts, croissants, pastries. Regular commercial muffins and quick breads like: Dunkin' Donuts® muffins or restaurant muffins, banana or nut breads or products made with shortening. Bisquick® and regular cake mixes.

Cereals with added fat like: Grape-Nuts Flakes®, Granola®, Cracklin' Oat Bran®

High-fat crackers like: Ritz®, clubs, Hi Hos®, Goldfish®, Town House®, Cheez-It®, Wheatsworth®, Nabisco American Classics®, Keebler Sun Toasted Wheats®

Milk and Milk Products
2-3 servings per day

Include

Skim milk
Evaporated skim milk
Nonfat dry milk
1% or 1/2% milk
Chocolate low fat milk
Instant malted milk
Hot cocoa mixes
Quick powder or syrup
Skim buttermilk
Nonfat yogurt
1 Tbsp. nondairy creamer
Non-fat Eagle Brand® Milk

(See Protein Foods for cheeses)

Avoid

Whole milk
2% milk (OK if you use only
  1 cup per day)
Cream
Half & half
Sour cream
Whipped cream
Evaporated 2% or whole milk
Eagle Brand® Condensed Milk
Milnot®
Powdered dry buttermilk

Miscellaneous

Include	Avoid
Healthy Choice® soups, Campbell's Healthy Request® soups, broth-type soups	Commercial cream soups
Spaghetti sauce like: Healthy Choice®, Ragu Today's Recipe®, Prince®, Weight Watchers®, and Hunts Tomato Sauce®	Prego Spaghetti Sauce® Chicken Tonight Sauces® Alfredo sauce White sauces
Vegetable pizza (thin crust with allowable amount of cheese)	
Frozen dinners like: Armour Classics Lite®, Budget Gourmet Lite & Healthy Dinners®, Eating Right®, Featherweight Healthy Recipes®, Health Valley®, Healthy Choice®, Stouffer's Right Course®, LeMenu Light®, Weight Watchers®	Other frozen dinners Most canned or boxed entrees
Cocoa powder	Solid chocolate
All regular microwave popcorn	
Regular granola bars	
All cheese or peanut butter snack crackers	

Nuts, Seeds, and Legumes

4-5 Servings per week

Include

Tree nuts, whose meat is plant material, contain no cholesterol and are high in unsaturated (good) fats; almonds, hazelnuts, macadamias, pecans, walnuts

Peanuts, a legume

2 Tbsp. peanut butter

2 Tbsp. seeds

1/2 cup dry beans

Avoid

None

Protein Foods

The word protein comes from the Greek word meaning "of first importance," a well-deserved name. Studies of protein show that the quality and quantity in a daily diet are of extreme importance. All protein molecules contain carbon, hydrogen, oxygen, and nitrogen. Proteins are large complex molecules made up of amino acids.

The cells of the body are composed mainly of protein, and tissue protein is constantly being broken down and must be replaced by dietary protein. Animal protein is the best quality protein because of its similarity to human protein tissue. Egg protein is considered to have the best amino acid pattern of any food; milk protein ranks next. Plant proteins are of lower quality because they lack one or more amino acids. When mixed together, however, plant proteins can provide high quality values.

Protein is broken down into each individual amino acid, which is then transported to the liver and then to the rest of the body cells. Some of the amino acids stay in the liver to replenish liver tissue or produce other plasma proteins. The rest are used by the body for tissue repairs. When energy from carbohydrates and fats is too low, protein can be used by the body as energy. If excess protein is consumed and can't be used for energy, some will be excreted in urine and feces and the balance will be stored as fat.

Because of the role protein plays in tissue building and repair, the needs of someone who is still growing or who is ill are greater than average. Persons recovering from surgery, burns, fever, or wound healing will use more protein than the average person of good health.

Sources of Protein

Lean meats
Poultry
Fish
Milk and milk products (except butter)
Eggs (the whites are mostly protein and contain no fat or cholesterol)
Legumes (peas, lentils, kidney beans, navy and pinto beans, peanuts, and garbanzos)

Luncheon meats have only about 1/2 to 2/3 of the protein of regular meats.

Include

Beef: USDA select grades of lean beef such as round, sirloin, flank, tenderloin, ground round (greater than 90% lean), pastrami

Pork: lean pork such as fresh ham, tenderloin, loin roast, loin chops, cured or boiled ham, Canadian bacon

Veal: all cuts are lean (chops, roasts, cutlets-unbreaded)

Poultry: skinless chicken, turkey, Cornish hen, ground turkey (greater than 90% lean), turkey ham, turkey pastrami

Eggs: egg whites (2 = 1 whole egg), egg substitutes, 4 egg yolks per week

Avoid

Beef: regular ground beef, ribs, chuck, steak (porterhouse, T-Bone), corned beef, prime cuts

Pork: spareribs, ground pork, pork sausage, pork steak and hocks, cracklings, bacon

Poultry: skin on poultry, domestic duck or goose, ground turkey less than 90% lean

Include (cont'd.)

Fish: all fresh and frozen fish, crab, lobster, scallops, shrimp, clams, oysters, tuna (canned in water), herring (pickled or smoked)

Cheese: 1% cottage cheese, ricotta, grated Parmesan, fat-free cheese, Limit the following to 1-2 times per week: Skim or part skim milk, cheeses such as: mozzarella, Kraft 2%, Farmers String Cheese®, Weight Watchers Natural Cheese®, Sargento's Light Cheese®, Alpine Lace®

Other: 95% fat-free luncheon meats, tofu, Harvest Burgers® (soy), Boca Burgers®, wild game such as venison

Avoid (cont'd.)

Fish: tuna canned in oil, any fried fish product, frozen breaded fish

Cheese: all regular cheeses such as American, blue, cheddar, Velveeta®, Monterey, jack, Swiss, cream cheese, Neufchatel

Other: other luncheon meats, liver, heart, kidney, sweetbreads, sausage, knockwurst, bratwurst, and frankfurters

- Choose 2-4 oz. at a meal (about the size of a deck of cards).

- Use low-fat cooking methods such as grilling, steaming, sauteing with nonstick spray, baking, or broiling. Drain all excess fat.

- Meat and cheeses should contain 5 grams of fat or less per ounce. Choose the leanest types, like turkey, chicken breast, fish, dried beans, etc.

- If you make meat salads or sandwiches, use light mayonnaise or mustard instead.

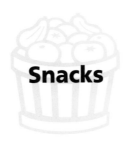

Snacks

Include	Avoid
Plain popcorn (hot air popped in a small amount of canola oil)	Impulse buying and eating
Some microwave popcorn (Orville Redenbacher Smart Pop®, Pop Secret Light®, Featherweight®, Weight Watchers®, Jolly Time Healthy Pop®)	
Pretzels	
Graham crackers (see other crackers in grain group)	
Rice cakes	
Baked tortilla chips (fat-free)	
Fruit rollups	
Health Valley Fat-free Fruit Bars®	
Fat-free potato chips	
Low-fat granola bars	

Sweets/Desserts

Think and plan ahead to have 5 or fewer
servings per week.

Include	Avoid
Candy: hard candies (gum drops, mints, butterscotch, etc.), gummy candies, chewing gum, circus peanuts, marshmallows	Chocolate, chocolate candy bars, caramels, peanut butter candies, fudge
Frosting: Fluffy white frosting mix (Betty Crocker® and Pillsbury®), Estee Frosting Mix®	Ready-to-spread frosting, butter cream frosting, decorator's frosting
Syrups: Hershey's® Chocolate Syrup, all pancake syrups (regular or sugar-free), corn syrup, molasses	Hot fudge
Cookies: animal crackers, fig bars, vanilla wafers, fat-free cookies (e.g., Entenmann's®, Archway®, Health Valley®, and Snackwell's®), Baker's Own® (Nabisco®), Famous Chocolate Wafers® (Nabisco®), Newtons®, gingersnaps, Social Tea Biscuits®, Archway Homestyle Molasses®	All regular commercial cookies
Cakes: angel food, Entenmann's Fat-free®, Sara Lee Free & Light®, Sara Lee Apple Crisp Cake®	All regular commercial cakes

Sweets/Desserts

Think and plan ahead to have 5 or fewer servings per week.

Include (cont'd.)	Avoid (cont'd.)
Cake Mixes: Pillsbury Gingerbread Mix®, Snackwell's Brownie Mix®	Regular cake mixes
Frozen Desserts: non-fat dairy desserts, Simple Pleasures®, frozen low-fat yogurt, sherbert, Popsicles®, Jello Pops®, Pudding Pops®, Colombo® and Dairy Queen® frozen yogurt	Regular ice cream, mocha mix, chocolate ice cream bars (regular or light), regular soft serve ice cream, milkshakes
Whipped Toppings: Fat-free Cool Whip®, Cool Whip Lite®, Dream Whip Topping Mix®, Featherweight® and Estee Whipped Topping Mix®	Regular Cool Whip® Reddi Whip®
Miscellaneous: puddings made from skim milk, Jello®, custard mix, Sara Lee Free & Light Strawberry Dessert®, Stouffer's Escalloped Apples®	Pie crust
Jam, jelly, preserves, apple butter, honey	
Sugar, artificial sweeteners	

Daily Guide to Sweetening
without Sugar

Type of sweetener and brand name	Major sweetening ingredient	Sweetness compared to sugar (amt. sweetener=amt. sugar)	Manufacturer's Suggested Uses
EQUAL® packets or tablets	Aspartame	1 packet = 2 tsp. 1 tablet = 1 tsp.	Table use, added to cold/hot foods (if added after cooking)
NUTRASWEET SPOONFUL®	Aspartame	1 tsp. = 1 tsp.	Table use, added to cold or non-baked recipes
SPRINKLE SWEET® packets	Saccharin	1 packet = 2 tsp.	Baking, cooking, and table use
SUGAR TWIN® regular & brown sugar replacements, powder, and packets	Saccharin	1 tsp. = 1 tsp. 1 Tbsp. = 1 Tbsp. 1 cup = 1 cup 1 packet = 2 tsp.	Baking, cooking, and table use
SWEET 10® liquid	Saccharin	1/8 tsp. (10 drops) = 1 tsp. 3/8 tsp. = 1 Tbsp. 2 Tbsp. = 1 cup	Table use and in cooking

Daily Guide to Sweetening
without Sugar

Type of sweetener and brand name	Major sweetening ingredient	Sweetness compared to sugar (amt. sweetener=amt. sugar)	Manufacturer's Suggested Uses
SWEET 'N LOW® Regular & brown sugar replacements, powder, and packets	Saccharin	1 tsp. = 1/4 cup 1 1/3 tsp. = 1/3 cup 2 tsp. = 1/2 cup 4 tsp. = 1 cup 1 packet = 2 tsp.	Baking, cooking, canning, and table use
SWEET MATE®	Aspartame	1 packet = 2 tsp.	Table use and added to cold or hot foods (if added after cooking)
SWEET ONE®	Acesulfame-K	1 packet = 2 tsp. 3 packets = 1/4 cup 4 packets = 1/3 cup 6 packets = 1/2 cup 12 packets = 1 cup	Table use, baking, and cooking

Vegetables

Include 4-5 daily servings

Include

Artichoke, asparagus, beans, bean sprouts, beets, broccoli, Brussels sprouts, cabbage, cauliflower, carrots, corn, eggplant, greens, kohlrabi, leeks, lima beans, mushrooms, okra, onions, peas, pea pods, peppers, potatoes, rutabaga, sauerkraut, spinach, squash, tomato, tomato/vegetable juice, tomato sauce (puree or paste), turnips, water chestnuts, yams, zucchini

Also, enchilada sauce, picant sauce, salsa, spaghetti sauce (Ragu's Today's Recipe® or Homestyle®), taco sauce

Avoid

Vegetables prepared in butter, cream, sour cream, or sauces

Fried vegetables and commercial salads with mayonnaise

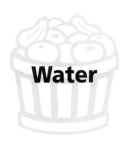

Water

There is always one common requirement with any diet, eight 8-oz. glasses of water per day! Ever wonder why? Next to oxygen, water is the body's most urgent need. It is more essential to life than food. Without water, nutrients are of no value to the body. A person can survive for weeks without food but only a few days without water.

Water makes up 1/2 to 3/4 of your body weight, depending on your age and the amount of body fat. Infants and children have a greater proportion of water than do older persons. Obese persons have less water than a lean person does.

Here's the percent of water contained in various parts of your body:

- 83% blood
- 73% lean muscle
- 25% fat
- 22% bone

What does water do for the body?

- Water helps to regulate body temperature, transports nutrients and other substances throughout the body, carries away waste, and moistens, lubricates, and cushions the body from injury. Water acts as a solvent to dissolve water-soluble vitamins.

- The body loses a total of about ten cups of water each day through exhaling, sweating, urinating, and bowel movements.

- Beverages containing caffeine or alcohol are dehydrating, so if you drink these, you need even more water to compensate.

- In the average diet foods can give the body about three to four cups of water per day.

- Want to have a better idea of how much water your body needs? Try this easy formula: 1-1$\frac{1}{2}$ milliliters (ml.) of water are needed daily per calorie. If you require 2,000 calories a day, you will need 2,000-3,000 ml. of water per day. 3,000 ml. would equal about 12 8-ounce glasses per day. This does not include making up for pop or coffee.

Drink to your health!

Other Beverages

Caffeine-Free coffee (or limit regular coffee to one cup per day)
Caffeine-Free tea
Caffeine-Free soft drinks
Juices
Lemonade
If you drink alcoholic beverages, do so in moderation and consult your physician.

What to Avoid and What to Choose

Are you making the correct food choices?

Product	Recommended servings	Choose	Avoid
Beans, Peas, etc.	Daily or substitute for two meals/week	Kidney, navy, lentils, red, northern, etc.	Canned refried beans
Soups	Bouillon, broth, and consomme, homemade soups with fat skimmed from broth, broth-based and tomato-based soups, homemade soups with skim milk, Healthy Request Cream Soup®	Cream soups, vichyssoise, chunky-style soups	
Breads	5 or more servings 1 serving equals: 1 slice bread 1/2 bagel 5-7 crackers 1 cup cold cereal 1/2 cup cooked cereal 1/2 cup cooked pasta 2 slices diet bread 1/2 cup rice	Most regular brands, wheat, white, rye, oat-meal, or oat bran types, English muffins, water bagels, buns, pita bread, tortillas (not fried), home-made quick breads, rice cakes, low fat Bisquick®, Special K® frozen waffles.	"buttercrust" or "cheese bread" egg bagels, croissants, doughnuts, sweet rolls, mixes yielding biscuits, waffles, etc.

Commercial biscuits, muffins, pancakes, and croissants that are not made with the recom-mended fats |

Product	Recommended servings	Choose	Avoid
Crackers	Saltines, graham, melba toast, Stoneground®, Wheatsworth®, matzoh, Rye Krisps®, Harvest Krisps®, Vegetable Krisps®	Cheese crackers and butter crackers, crackers made with palm oil, palm kernel oil, or coconut oil	
Snacks		Popcorn (air popped, microwave), pretzels, fig bars, graham crackers (2 per serving), animal crackers (8 per serving), rice cakes	Buttered popcorn, most microwave popcorn, potato chips, corn chips, onion rings, snacks with "sugar" listed as the first or second ingredient on label
Cereal		All types except those in Avoid column; 10 grams of sugar or less per serving	Granola (or any with coconut oil), hot cereal with cream added, brands with sugar listed as first or second on label
Pasta		All types made without egg yolk, including macaroni, spaghetti, noodles, and rice	Pasta and rice prepared with whole eggs, cream sauce, or high fat cheese
Tofu	6 grams of fat/ 3 oz. regular		

Product	Recommended servings	Choose	Avoid
Meat and Meat substitute Red Meat, 3 times per week only	Limit to 6 oz. per day, 3 oz. (size of deck of cards)	Trim all visible fat. Select lean cuts, such as round steak, sirloin tip, tenderloin, chipped beef, ground round, center cut ham, Canadian bacon, tenderloin, loin chops, veal (cubed, shoulder, or sirloin), Healthy Choice® hot dog/bologna	Organ meats, "Prime" grade, all rib cuts, sausage, frankfurters, bacon, regular luncheon meats, Spam®, tongue
Poultry		Skinless chicken breast, Cornish hen and turkey with skin removed, 97-100% lean ground turkey breast	Poultry skin, poultry luncheon meats, duck, goose
Eggs		All egg whites and egg substitutes (Egg Beaters®). May have 3 egg yolks per week if desired	Fried eggs
Peanut Butter	2 Tbsp. once a week, if desired	2 Tbsp. replaces one oz. of meat, old fashion and regular types	

Product	Recommended servings	Choose	Avoid
Seafood		All fresh and frozen fish, tuna canned in water, cold scallops Limit the use of shellfish to one 3 oz. serving per week (lobster, shrimp, and crab), haddock, perch, pollack, trout, halibut, salmon	Fish canned in oil Caviar Fried fish
Wild Game		Venison, rabbit, squirrel, pheasant, without skin	
Vegetables and Fruit	6 servings/day 1 serving = 1/2 cup cooked or 1 cup raw	All are acceptable if plain baked, boiled, and mashed potatoes, frozen hash browns	Avocado, coconut, guacamole, fruits in heavy syrup, vegetables packed in a butter, cheese, or cream sauce, fried vegetables, French fries, Tator Tots®
Fats and Oils Vegetable Oils	6 servings/day All oils have 5 grams of fat per teaspoon	Sunflower, corn, soybean, sesame, canola, peanut, and olive, 1 serving = 1 tsp.	Coconut, palm, palm kernel, and solid vegetable shortening, i.e., Crisco®, lard, beef tallow

Product	Recommended servings	Choose	Avoid
Margarines	1 serving = 1 tsp. (As a general guide, select margarine with liquid oil listed as the first ingredient)	Fleischmann's Light®, Promise Ultra®, Shedd's Butter Buds®. Molly McButter®	Butter, lard, bacon drippings, ham hocks, salt pork, meat fat, gravy made from meat drippings
Salad Dressing	(1 serving = 1 Tbsp.) Fat-free, Non-fat Dressing	French, Italian, oil and vinegar, sweet 'n sour, Light Miracle Whip®, Weight Watchers Mayonnaise®, salad dressing, with 10 calories or less per Tbsp.	Cream dressings such as blue cheese, Thousand Island, buttermilk dressings, mayonnaise, regular Miracle Whip®
Frozen Desserts	1/3-1/2 cup = serving; 3 gm. fat or less per 4 oz. serving	Sugar-free popsicles, fudgesicles, sugar-free frozen yogurt, sugar-free ice milk, TCBY® sugar-free frozen yogurt	Ice cream (soft serve or hard pack) Ice milk made with whole milk
Desserts	May have 2 regular desserts per week from allowed list	Sugar-free gelatin, angel food cake, Duncan Hines® white cake mix, sugar-free pudding, fruit ices, popsicles, sorbet, homemade desserts if made with approved ingredients, DQ Fudge Bars® made with Nutra Sweet®, TCBY® sugar-free non-fat yogurt	Desserts containing cream, whole milk, solid chocolate, cream cheese, coconut, carob, Store bought cakes, pies, cookies, and mixes

Product	Recommended servings	Choose	Avoid
Others		Avocado (1 serving = 1/8 medium) Olives (1 serving = 10 small or 5 large) All seeds and most nuts (1 serving = 1 Tbsp.), 5 grams of fat	Cashews, macadamias, pistachios
Miscellaneous		Decaffeinated tea and coffee, herbal tea, caffeine-free, sugar free diet carbonated beverages, Cary's® syrup, herbs, spices, catsup, mustard, unsweetened fruit drinks, dry cocoa powder, sugar-free jelly, sugar-free hot cocoa, sugar-free hard candies, Crystal Light®, Equal®, Sweet One®, Sweet 'n Low®, Nutra Sweet®	Regular coffee, regular tea, gravies, butter sauces, chocolate, coconut, regular pop, alcohol, sugar, jelly, jam, honey, molasses, syrup, marshmallows, jelly beans, gum drops, licorice, mints, and peanuts

Grocery Guide

Beans
Canned (no salt added)
Canned (without fat; rinse salt off)
Dried (any)
Fat-free refried beans (any)

Bread (whole grain)
(1 gram of fat or less/ per serving)
Aunt Millie's 100% Whole Wheat®
Brownberry Natural Wheat®
Pepperidge Farm®
(100% Stoneground Whole Wheat,
Honey Oat, Crunchy Grains)
Southern Country 100% Whole Wheat®

Butter (non-fat substitutes)
Butter Buds®
Butter Buds® sprinkles
Molly McButter® (butter, sour
cream, cheese, garlic butter)

Cereals (non-oat)
(Whole grain, 3 grams or more
of fiber, 2 grams or less of fat;
8 grams or less of sucrose and
other sugars, unless contains
dried fruit, in which case may
contain up to 14 grams; no nuts,
sulfured fruit or artificial
color/flavor/sweetener; no
coconut/palm oil)
Flavorite Bran Flakes®
Raisin Bran®
Nutty Nuggets®
General Mills Fiber One®
Multigrain Cheerios®
General Mills Wheaties®
Total®

Total Raisin Bran®
Healthy Choice®
All varieties Kellogg's
Complete Wheat Bran Flakes®
Kellogg's All-Bran®
Bran Buds®
Kellogg's Frosted Mini-Wheats®
Apple Raisin Crisp®
Meuslix®
Kellogg's Nutri-Grain Wheat®,
Wheat and Raisin®
Kellogg's Mini-Wheats®: Raisin,
Strawberry, Blueberry, Apple
Cinnamon
Multigrain Chex®
Nabisco 100% Bran®
Nabisco Cream of Wheat®
Nabisco Shredded Wheat®
Nabisco Frosted Wheat Squares®
Nabisco Shredded Wheat N' Bran®
Post Honey Nut Shredded Wheat®
Post Fruit & Fiber®
Post Grape-Nuts and Flakes®
Post Bran Flakes®
Post Raisin Bran®
Post Shredded Wheat 'n Bran®
Quaker Shredded Wheat®
Multi-Bran Chex®
Wheat bran (any)
Wheat germ (any)
Whole Grain Wheat Chex®

Cereals (oat)
(Oat bran, whole oats, or whole
oat flour listed as first ingredient;
3 grams or more of fiber; 2 grams
or less fat; no palm or coconut
oil; no artificial color, flavor, or

sweetener; 8 grams or less
sucrose and other sugars, unless
contains dried fruit, in which
case may have up to 14 grams;
no nuts or sulfured fruits)
Oatmeal, plain (any)
Oat bran, plain (any)
General Mills Instant Total Oatmeal®:
regular flavor
Healthy Valley Fat-free Granola®
Healthy Valley Oat Bran O's®
Healthy Valley Oat Bran Flakes®
Healthy Valley Fruit and Nut Oat
Bran Flakes®
Kellogg's Common Sense Oat Bran®
Kellogg's Common Sense Oat Bran
with Raisins®
Quaker Extra®: regular flavor,
raisin & cinnamon
Quaker Toasted Oatmeal Squares®
Quaker Oatbran®
Quaker Instant Oatmeal®: Regular,
Cinnamon & Spice, Maple &
Brown Sugar

Cheese (low fat, less than 5 grams fat/ounce)

Fat-free
Borden's Fat-free Singles®
Flavorite Fat-free Singles®
Frigo No-fat Ricotta®
Healthy Choice Fat-free Cream
Cheese®, string cheese, shredded
Cheese, block processed cheese
Kraft Philadelphia Non-fat Cream
Cheese®
Kraft Reduced-fat Grated
Parmesan®
Kraft Free Singles®/Kraft Fat-free
Shredded®
Light N' Lively Free Cottage Cheese®

Meijer® Fat-free dairy products
Weight Watchers Fat-free Slices®

Less than 5 grams Fat/Ounce
Alouette Light Spread®
Borden Lite-Line® slices (any)
Cheese-Wiz Light®
Cottage cheese, low fat (any)
County Line Advantage® (any)
County Line Light Shredded
Cheese®
Healthy Choice®-low fat (any)
Kraft® 2% milk (any)
Kraft Philadelphia Light Cream
Cheese®
Kraft Light 'n Lively® Process
Cheese Product
Parmesan (any) in small amounts
Part Skim or Low-fat ricotta
cheese
Part Skim mozzarella or string
cheese
Sargento-Lights®
Weight Watchers® American flavor
Process Cheese Product
Veggie Slices® (any)
Veggie Shreds®
Velveeta-Light®
Yoder's Light Ricotta Cheese®
Yoder's Shredded Cheddar®

Chicken & Turkey
Butterball Chicken Requests®
Butterball Lean Turkey Burgers®
Butterball Oven Roasted Turkey
Breast®
Butterball Seasoned Chicken®
Breast (teriyaki, lemon, Italian)
Louis Rich Oven Roasted Breast of
Turkey® (regular and no salt added)

Canned
Valley Fresh White Chicken® in water
Swanson White Chicken® in water
Sweet Sue Chicken® in water
Hormel Chicken® in water

Cocoa & Chocolate
Carnation Fat-free Cocoa®
Hershey's Cocoa® (low-fat substitute for baking chocolate)
Hershey's Fat-free Dutch Chocolate®
Swiss Miss Fat-free Sugar Free Cocoa®
Swiss Miss Diet®
Swiss Miss Fat-free French Vanilla®
Swiss Miss Fat-free Marshmallow Lovers®

Coffee
Any brands which are 97% and higher decaffeinated

Cookies (select cookies with 1 grams of fat or less/serving)
Archway Fat-free Oatmeal Raisin Cookies®
Entemann's Fat-free Cookies®
Gingersnaps
Graham crackers, Low-fat
Nabisco Fig Newtons®, Fat-free (any)
Snackwell's® low-fat and Fat-free varieties
Weight Watchers Oatmeal Raisin and Fruit-filled Cookies®

Low-fat Cookies (more than 1 gram of fat/serving)
Keebler Reduced Fat Fudge Stripe Cookies®
Reduced Fat Oreo®
Reduced Fat Chips Ahoy!®

Reduced Fat Vanilla Wafers®
Snackwell's
Teddy Grahams

Crackers/Snacks (try to use whole grain or mostly whole grain; monitor portions of all free items)

Fat-free
Baked Ruffles® (any)
Cracker Jack®, Fat-free
Crunch n' Munch®, Fat-free
Keebler Zesta®, Fat-free
Nabisco Premium®, Fat-free
Rice cakes (any)
Pringles®, Fat-free
Snackwell's® Fat-free Crackers® (any)
Sunshine Krispy® Fat-free
WOW Chips® (any)

Less than 2 grams of Fat/Serving
Animal crackers
General Mills Crisp Baked Bugles®
Melba toast (any)
Mike-Sell's Reduced Fat Potato Chips®
Nabisco Harvest Crisp-Orchard Crisp®, Garden Crisps®
Nabisco Oysterettes®, Premium Soups® and Oyster Crackers®
Nabisco Zweiback Toast®
Snackwell's Snack Crackers®
Tostitos Baked Tortilla Chips®

Crackers
Keebler Reduced Fat Club®
Keebler Reduced Fat Town House®
Nabisco Air Crisps®
Nabisco Reduced Fat Cheese Nips®
Nabisco Reduced Fat Triscuits®
Nabisco Reduced Fat Wheat Thins®
Nabisco Reduced Fat Better Cheddar®

Nabisco Reduced Fat Ritz®
Sunshine Reduced Fat Cheez-It®

Croutons
Pepperidge Farm Fat-free Caesar®
Rothbury Farms Fat-free Seasoned
   Croutons®

Eggs/Egg Substitutes
Better'n Eggs®
Deb El® (Just Whites, Scramblettes®)
   (dry mix)
Egg whites
Egg Beaters®

Fish
Canned
Chicken of the Sea Tuna® in water,
   50% less salt
Polar Crab Meat®
Salmon (any, except boneless or
   smoked)
Star Kist Select Chunk Light Tuna
   in Spring Water®, Low Sodium®,
   Low-fat
Tuna packed in water (any)

Fresh
From unpolluted waters, freshwater
fish such as trout from mountain
streams, saltwater fish such as
flounder, sole haddock, halibut,
cod, ocean perch, pollock, grouper,
snapper, turbot, salmon, tuna

Highest in Omega-3 Fatty Acids
Mackerel (Atlantic), herring
(Atlantic), bluefish, salmon (red),
sardines

Frozen
Gorton's Grilled Fillets®

Harvest of the Sea-Cooked,
   Frozen Shrimp®
Louis Kemp® Imitation Crab,
   Scallops, Lobster
Mrs. Paul's Grilled Fillets®
Van de Kamp's Grilled Salmon and
   Tuna®
Van de Kamp's Krisp and Healthy
   Breaded Fish®
Wakefield® snow crab meat

Bacon
Butterball Turkey Bacon® (2 grams
   of fat/slice)
Jenni-O Extra Lean Turkey Bacon®
   (0.5 grams of fat/slice)

Sausage
Butterball® Fat-free Polaska
   Kielbasa and Smoked Sausage
Eckrich® Fat-free Sausage: Kielbasa
   and smoked Healthy Choice
   Breakfast Sausage
Healthy Choice Low-fat Polaska
   Kielbasa®

Ground Meat (2 grams of fat or
   less/ounce)
Butterball 97% Fat-free Extra Lean
   Ground Turkey®
Healthy Choice® Extra Lean Turkey
   and Hamburger
Deli-ground turkey breast

Meat Substitutes and
Soy Products
Amy's Veggie Burgers®
Boca Meatless Tenders and
   Breakfast Links®
Boca Burger® (any)
Garden Burger® (any)
Green Giant Vegetable Protein®
   products (any)

Harmony Farms Soy Burgers®
Morningstar Farms® meat products
Naturally Preferred Fat-free Soy
    Milk®
Silk Soy Milk®, Low-fat
Smart Deli Meatless Fat-free Slices®
Soya Kaas Soy Cheese®
Tofu Rella Soy Cheese®
Yves Soy Protein® products (any)
West Soy Light and Non-fat Soy
    Milk®
West Soy Juice Soy Burger®
Worthington® meatless products
Veggie Cheese® products
Zen Don Soy Milk®

Milk

Borden Eagle Bran Fat-free®
Sweetened Condensed Milk®
Carnation Low-fat and Fat-free
    Evaporated Milk®
Carnation Fat-free Coffee-Mate®
Farm Rich Fat-free Non-dairy
    Creamer®
International Delights Fat-free
    Creamers®
Lactaid Lactose Reduced Non-fat
    Milk®
Non-fat dry powdered milk (any)
Fat-free milk
Low-fat milk
Pet Light Evaporated Skimmed
    Milk®
SACO Cultured Buttermilk Blend®

Ketchup/Mustard

Ketchup
Heinz Tomato Ketchup®-no salt
    added

Mustard
Any without added oil

Lowest in Sodium
French's Classic Yellow Mustard®
Plochman's Yellow Mustard®
Gulden's Spicy Brown Mustard®
Flavorite Prepared Mustard®

Nuts

Although nuts are "good fats," they
contain 90% of their calories from
fat, therefore limit intake.

Oils (unsaturated; not hydrogenated)
    All contain 12-14 grams fat/Tbsp.,
    so use sparingly.
Crisco®
Mazola®
Wesson 100% Corn Oil®
Olive, preferably extra-virgin (any)
Smucker's Baking Healthy 100%
    Fat-free®
Wesson®
Mazola®: Canola®, and Vegetable
    Oil Blend®

Pancakes/Waffles (partly whole
    grain)
Aunt Jemima®
Aunt Jemima Low-fat Waffles and
    Pancakes®
Bisquick Reduced Fat Mix®
Downyflake Crisp and Healthy Waffles®
Eggo Fat-free Waffles®
Eggo Low-fat Nutri-Grain Waffles®
Hodgson Mill Whole Wheat® or
    Buckwheat Pancake Mix®
Mrs. Butterworth's® complete,
    buttermilk complete
Pepperidge Farm Whole Wheat
    Pancake Mix®
Pillsbury, Hungry Jack Buttermilk
    Complete Mix®
Lite syrups (any)

Pasta

Chef Boyardee 99% Fat-free Beef Ravioli® (high in sodium)
Fresh or dry pasta, unfilled (any, preferably whole wheat)
Kraft Light Pasta Salad®
Mueller's Yolk Free Noodle Style Pasta®
No Yolks®
Pasta Roni® (any) prepared using less fat instructions

Peanut Butter (no hydrogenated oil; no sugar)

(contains 6 grams fat/Tbsp, should be limited)
Jiff Reduced Fat®
Peter Pan Reduced Fat®
Skippy Reduced Fat®
Smucker's Natural Reduced Fat®

Soup

Campbell's 98% Fat-free® soups
Campbell's Low Sodium Chicken Broth®
Campbell's Low-fat Ramen Noodles®
Fat-free canned broth or bouillon
Healthy Choice® soups
Lipton® dry soup mixes
Progresso® (any without cream, if diluted with low sodium chicken broth)
Swanson Natural Goodness Clear Chicken Broth® (less salt)
Swanson Clear Vegetable Broth®
Uncle Ben's Hearty Soups Black Bean® (high in sodium)

Sour Cream/Dips (lower fat)

Breakstone's Fat-free Sour Cream®
Prairie Farms Fat-free Sour Cream®
Guilt Free Sour Cream®
Land O' Lakes® Light Non-fat sour cream/dips
Light 'n Lively Fat-free Sour Cream®
Real Dairy Non-fat Sour Cream®
T. Marzetti's® Fat-free and light dips

Spaghetti Sauce (under 700 mg. sodium; under 30% calories from fat)

Classico®: Mushroom & Olive, Tomato & Basil
Del Monte Traditional with Green Peppers and Mushrooms®
Five Brothers®: Tomato & Basil, Marinara
DiGiorno Fat-free®
Healthy Choice®
Hunt's No Added Sugar®
Muir Glen Organic Fat-free Spaghetti Sauce®
Prego®: Garden Variety and Three Cheese)
Weight Watcher's Spaghetti Sauce with Mushrooms®
Weight Watcher's Spaghetti Sauce Flavored with Meat®
Newman's Own®: Marinara, Tomato Peppers & Spices

Spices/Seasonings

Blends

Mrs. Dash® (any)
Old El Paso 40% Less Sodium Taco Seasoning Mix®

Individual Spices

All-any brand
Durkee Smart Seasoning® (any)

Tea

Decaffeinated tea (any)

Tortillas
Fat-free (any)

Tofu (1 gram or less fat/3 oz.)
Mori-Nu Lite Tofu®

Vegetables
Canned (no added salt or rinse off surface salt)
Fresh (any)
Frozen (any without sauces/ seasoning packets)

Vegetable Juices (no salt added)
Campbell's Low Sodium Tomato Juice®
V8 Juice®, No Salt Added
Hollywood 100% Pure Carrot Juice®
Hunt's All Natural Tomato Juice® (no salt added)

Vegetable Sprays
Country Crock Butter Flavored Fat-free Spray®
PAM® or any other brand (any)
Weight Watcher's Butter Spray®
Canola oil cooking spray®

Vinegar
Any (balsamic vinegar can be used as a salad dressing)

Yogurt
Fat-free
Breyer's® Fat-free
Dannon Light Non-fat®
Light 'n Lively Free®
Meijer® Non-fat®
TCBY® Non-fat®
Yoplait Fat-free Light®
Yoplait Fat-free Fruit on Top®

Low-fat
TCBY® Low-fat
Yoplait 98% Fat-free®
Dannon Light 'N Fit®
Dannon® (any)
Breyer's® (any)

Frozen Dinners and Entrees
(All items have values for sodium and fat as shown below)

Sodium
Entrees: 800 mg. or less
Dinners: 900 mg. or less

Fat
Entrees: 30% or less kcal from fat
Dinners: 30% or less kcal from fat

Sodium Restriction
Most frozen dinners will be high in sodium. Choose dinners which are low in sodium and work them into your daily sodium budget.

Budget Gourmet Low-fat Meals®
Healthy Choice Meals®
Michelina Low-fat Meals®
Stouffer's Lean Cuisine®
Uncle Ben's Rice Bowls® (high in sodium)
Weight Watcher's Smart Ones®

Flour (whole grain)
Whole wheat
Whole rye
Cornmeal (if not "bolted" or "degerminated")

Fruit
Canned or bottled in water, juice, or extra-light syrup
Del Monte Light®

Dried (no sulfates): raisins, currants, dates, prunes, cranberries, and cherries
Fresh (any)
Frozen (any without sugar)
Liberty Gold Light®
Libby's Lite®
Natural applesauce

Fruit Juice
Fresh, canned or bottled, brick-packed, or frozen 100% juice
Libby's Juicy Juice®
Minute Maid Calcium Fortified 100% Orange Juice®
Old Orchard 100% Juice®: Apple Blackberry, Cranberry Blend, Apple Peach Mango
Tropicana Plus Calcium 100% Orange Juice®

Game Meats
Rabbit, pheasant, deer, etc.

Gelatin
Knox®, unflavored
Sugar-free (any)

Granola/Granola Bars
Kellogg's Nutri Grain Bars/Twists®
Nabisco Fruit 'N Grain Bars®
Quaker Low Fat Chewy Granola Bars®: Apple Berry, Oatmeal Raisin, S'mores

Gravy (1 gram or less per serving)
Durkee Gravy Mix®
Flavorite Brand Gravy Mix®
Franco-American Fat-free Gravy®: Beef, Chicken, and Turkey
French's Gravy Mix®

Heinz Fat-free Gravy®
Heinz Homestyle Gravy®
Knorr Gravy Mix®
Pepperidge Farm® gravies

Ice Milk/Frozen Yogurt/Juice Bars/Sorbet
(no artificial colors, flavors, or sweeteners; no coconut or cream)

Fat Free
Atz's Fat-free Frozen Yogurt®
Ben and Jerry's No-fat®
Bordon Non-fat®
Breyer's Fat-free®
Dole Fruit Juice Bars®
Edy's Fat-free and Non-fat desserts
Edy's Fruit Bars®
Guilt Free Sugar-free Ice Cream®
Juice bars (any without coconut or cream)
Kemp's Non-fat Frozen Yogurt®
Non-fat fudge bars
Popsicles®
Sherbet
Sorbet (any)
Weight Watcher's Fat-free®
Welch's Fruit Juice Bars®

Less than 2 gram fat per 1/2 cup
Atz's® frozen desserts (sugar-free and low-fat)
Ben and Jerry's Light®: Banana Strawberry, Cherry Garcia, Blueberry Cheesecake
Breyer's®
Edy's® Low-fat
Healthy Choice 98% Fat-free®
Homemade Low-fat Ice Cream®
Kemp's Sugar-free Frozen Yogurt®
Velvet Frozen Yogurt®
Velvet Frozen Dessert Light Sugar-free®

Sugar-free
Ice Milk Toppings
Hershey's Lite Chocolate Syrup®
Hershey's Sundae Syrup, Fat-free®
Hershey's Strawberry Syrup, Fat-free®
Hershey's Fat-free Hot Fudge®
Heath Sundae Syrup English Toffee, Fat-free®
Mrs. Richard's Fat-free Hot Fudge and Caramel Fudge®
Smucker's Fat-free Syrup®: caramel, butterscotch
Smucker's Topping®, Fat-free (any)
Smucker's Fat-free Light Topping Hot Fudge®

Other Toppings
Cool Whip Fat-free Topping®

Jam (no artificial colorings)
Low in Sugar
Knott's Berry Farm Light Fruit Spread®
Smucker's Light Sugar-free® (any)
Smucker's Low Sugar®

No added sugar
Knott's Berry Farm Light Fruit Spread®
Polander All Fruit®
Smucker's Simply Fruit Spreads®

Margarine (try to select 6 grams of fat or less/tablespoon)
(At least twice as much polyunsaturated as saturated fat; liquid polyunsaturated vegetable oil heading the list of ingredients)

Fat-fee (tub)
Promise Ultra Fat-free®
Fleischmann's Fat-free®
I Can't Believe It's Not Butter Fat-free®

Less 6 grams of fat/tablespoon
Blue Bonnet® Lower-fat margarine
Brummel & Brown® margarine
Butter Buds® tub margarine
Country Crock Light®
Fleischmann's® Lower-fat tub or stick
I Can't Believe It's Not Butter Light®
Mazola Extra Light®
Parkay Light Spread® in the tub
Promise Margarine Extra Light® and Ultra Light®
Smart Beat Margarine/Trans Free®
Smart Balance Light®
Weight Watcher's Extra Light®
Weight Watcher's Country Cottage® (blue or green label)
Weight Watcher's Sodium Free Light Margarine®

Pump Spray
I Can't Believe It's Not Butter®
Country Crock®
Parkay®

Spreads
Benecol® and Benecol Light Spread®
Take Control®

Mayonnaise Sandwich Spreads (lower in calories; no artificial coloring)
Hellmann's Low-fat Mayonnaise®
Hellmann's Reduced Fat Tarter Sauce®

Kraft Free Mayonnaise®
Kraft Free Tarter Sauce®
Kraft Miracle Whip Fat-free®
Kraft Miracle Whip Light®
Weight Watcher's Fat-free
    Mayonnaise®

Meat (lowest fat cuts-choose from select grade, if possible)

Beef
Eye of Round (roast or steak)
Ground Beef cuts with loin or
    round in their name are the leanest
    (ground round or ground sirloin)
Round Tip (roast)
Sirloin
Tenderloin (also called filet mignon
    or fillet steak)
Top Loin (also called New York
    Strip, Club, Delmonico, or Strip
    Steak)
Top Round

Lamb
Blade Chops
Foreshank
Loin Chops
Rack (Rib)
Shank Half Leg Roast
Sirloin Roast

Pork
Canadian Bacon
Whole Leg
Leg, Rump Half
Loin (Center Loin Roast or Chop)
Boneless Ham, trimmed of visible
    fat (fresh cooked, deli sliced,
    pre-sliced, canned)

Veal
Arm Steak
Blade Steak
Cutlet
Loin Chop
Rib Roast
Sirloin Chop

Hot Dogs
Ball Park Fat-free®
Ball Park Lite Franks®
Butterball Fat-free®
Eckrich Fat-free®
Healthy Choice 97% Fat-free®
Oscar Meyer Fat-free®

Lunch Meats (less than 1 gram of fat per serving; deli meats con tain less sodium)
Butterball Fat-free®
Carl Budding Lean Slices, Turkey
    99% Fat-free®
Eckrich Fat-free®
Healthy Choice®
Hillshire Farms 97%-99% Fat-free
    Deli Meats®
Hormel Light and Lean®
Louis Rich Free®
Oscar Meyer Fat-free®
Sara Lee Homeroast®
Thorne Apple Valley® 97% Fat-free
    Turkey and Ham

Plan Ahead for Eating Out

- Try not to wait until the last minute to eat out. If you can decide what you want beforehand, you may avoid temptations at the restaurant.

- Be the first to order if you tend to be influenced by others.

- Ask questions when ordering:

    How is this fixed? Could I have it baked?

    Will you put the dressing or sauce on the side? (Then dip your fork into the dressing before stabbing salad.)

    Will you please leave off the sour cream, butter, or cheese sauce.

    Can I order a la carte, or can an appetizer be ordered as a main course?

    Do you have smaller portions or can we share an entrée?

    Can I have a doggie bag?

- Control portions of salad dressing, margarine, chips, and quick breads, such as muffins.

- Take your own salad dressing or Butterbuds.

- To avoid overeating and/or tempting foods, concentrate on the non-food related pleasures of eating out:

    Not having to cook.

    Not having to wash dishes.

    Relaxed conversation with friends or spouse.

    Time away from the children or time with the children.

    Pleasant atmosphere.

Select from the Menu When Eating Out

Appetizer: Fresh fruit, raw vegetables, fruit or vegetable juices, radishes, raw or steamed clams or oysters, bouillon, consommé or broth-type soup, broiled shrimp.

Avoid patés, sauces, cold cuts, quiche, fried vegetables or fried shrimp, fried cheese.

Entrée: Broiled or roasted lean beef, veal, lamb, chicken, turkey; broiled or poached fish, shrimp, crabmeat, stir-fried Oriental chicken and vegetable dishes, vegetable pizza, meatless spaghetti with Parmesan cheese, bean burrito without cheese, chicken fajita.

Avoid cream sauces, dressing, gravies, breaded or fried meats, casseroles, stews, steaks, sausage, processed luncheon meats, bacon, stir-fried dishes containing fried meats, or nuts.

Salads: Tossed salads with vinegar, lemon, or dressing on the side; raw vegetables, fruit salads, cottage cheese, relishes; may use small amounts of avocado or sunflower seeds.

Avoid creamy dressings, bacon, croutons, egg yolks, coleslaw, salad with mayonnaise, cheese crackers.

Vegetables: All steamed, broiled, stir-fried; baked potato-plain.

Avoid butter, sauces, breading, creamed, au gratin, sauteed.

Breads: Hard rolls, French or Italian breads, bread sticks without butter, crackers.

Avoid muffins, cornbread, croissants, biscuits, butter rolls, garlic toast, sweet rolls, Danish, coffee cake, doughnuts; use butter or margarine sparingly.

Desserts: Fruit ices, sherbet, angel food cake, fresh fruit, low fat yogurt, gelatin.

Avoid pies, cakes, puddings, ice cream, whipped cream, cookies, custards, pastries.

Beverages: Fruit juices, decaffeinated coffee, tea, soda, club soda, mineral water, skim milk, water; limit alcohol to one serving of dry wine or light beer or mixed drink, if any.

Avoid chocolate milk, shakes, ice cream drinks.

Fats: Use margarine or salad dressing sparingly.

Avoid fried foods, butter, sour cream, gravies, cream sauces.

Fast-Food Choices

On a typical day, one out of five people in the U.S. will line up at the fast-food counter. In fact, according to research, more than half the meals purchased outside the home come from fast-food restaurants. This is the most challenging restaurant from which to select proper foods. Although fast-food restaurants are becoming more attentive to nutrition concerns, ideally this is not your best choice and should not be a frequent one.

When the choice is fast-food:

1. Choose small or "junior" portions or single hamburgers without cheese. Avoid the "extra" or "super."

2. Scrape off or request burgers and grilled chicken without excess dressing, butter, tartar sauce, and mayonnaise.

3. Avoid fast-food desserts and French fries. Plain baked potatoes and whole-grain sandwich buns have been added to "light menus," such as Wendy's. Frozen yogurt is an acceptable dessert.

4. Many establishments have chicken and fish dishes that are grilled, broiled, or steamed:

    Long John Silver's: baked fish dinner

    Hardee's: grilled chicken sandwich, grilled chicken salad, small cone

    Burger King: BK Broiler (request without ranch sauce), bagel (without cream cheese), garden salad

    McDonald's: plain hamburger, chunky chicken salad, side salad, grilled chicken

    Arby's: roast beef, no cheese

Taco Bell: soft taco-steak or light chicken

Subway: Lite menu choices, turkey breast salad

5. While fish and chicken may seem to be lower-fat selections, avoid the fried versions. Chicken McNuggets and Filet-O-Fish sandwiches provide more fat calories than a Quarter Pounder (which is also a bad choice).

6. If you must order deep-fried foods, take off the breading, skin, or other coating.

7. Fast-food roast beef usually has less fat than a hamburger, if it is available.

8. Request juice, low-fat milk, or diet soda instead of shakes and whole milk.

9. Don't sabotage your salad with rich, fatty dressings, bacon bits, cheddar cheese, and butter-fried croutons.

10. Beware, one small ladle of dressing holds 4 tablespoons, or up to 350 calories. Watch portions on fat sources.

11. With a tomato sauce base, mozzarella cheese, and a flour-baked crust (not pan fried), pizza offers a fairly low-fat package. Avoid the processed meats and extra cheese. Good choices are Domino's cheese and vegetable or Papa John's cheese and vegetable.

12. Balance out an occasional fast-food meal by eating fruits, vegetables, and whole grains at the day's other meals.

Fast-food: Music to Your Ears!

Fast-food can fit into a heart healthy lifestyle. The following items contain less than 12 grams of fat. Stop and think before you choose; try to make the best choice possible.

Arby's®
Junior Roast Beef (10g)
Light Roast Chicken Deluxe (7g)
Light Roast Turkey Deluxe (6g)
Light Roast Beef Deluxe (10g)
Chef Salad (no dressing) (9.5g)
Roast Chicken Salad (7g)
Garden Salad (no dressing) (5.2g)

Burger King®
Hamburger (10g)
BK Broiler Chicken Sandwich (without sauce or cheese) (8g)
6 Chicken Tenders (12g)
Broiled Chicken Salad (with Weight Watcher's Creamy Ranch) (4g)
Garden Salad (5g)

Chick-Fil-A®
Hearty Breast of Chicken Soup (3g)
Char-grilled Chicken Sandwich (5g)
Char-grilled Chicken Salad (2g)
Tossed Salad with Light Dressing (1g)
Carrot Raisin Salad (5g)
Ice Dream, small (5g)

Dairy Queen®
Frozen Yogurt Cone (1g)
Frozen Yogurt Cup (0.5g)
Breeze (strawberry) (2g)
BBQ Beef Sandwich (4g)
Grilled Chicken Sandwich (no toppings) (8g)
Side Salad (no dressing) (0g)

Fazoli's®
Minestrone Soup (3g)
Bread stick (no butter) (1g)
Baked Ziti (12g)
Small Spaghetti with Tomato or Meat Sauce (8g)
Double Slice Cheese Pizza (11g)
Garden Salad (with 1 Tbsp. Low Calorie Dressing) (2g)

Hardee's®
Grilled Chicken Sandwich (10g)
Reg. Roast Beef (11g)
Ham and Cheese (12g)
Hamburger (10g)
3 Pancakes (with syrup) (2g)
Cool Twist Cone (2g)

Long John Silver's®
Clam Chowder (6g)
Ocean Chef Salad (5g)
Rice Pilaf (3g)
Baked Fish with Lemon (with breadcrumbs) (3g)
Baked Cod (no butter) (1g)
Corn on the Cob (0g)
Green Beans (1g)

McDonald's®
Apple Bran/Blueberry Muffin (3g)
Cheerios/Wheaties with 1% Milk (1g)
English Muffin w/margarine (5g)
Hot Cakes/Syrup (12g)
Chunky Chicken Salad (4 Tbsp. vinaigrette dressing) (7g)
Chicken Fajita (8g)

McDonald's® (cont'd.)

Hamburger (9g)

McLean Deluxe (no sauce or cheese) (9g)

Frozen Yogurt Cone (2g)

Low-fat Milkshake (5g)

Pizza Hut®

2 slices medium, thin, or hand tossed crust, vegetable, cheese, Canadian bacon, BBQ Chicken (22g)

Plain Bread stick (with pizza sauce) (2g)

Subway®

(all ordered without oil or mayonnaise)

4" Round Turkey, Ham (6g)

6" Ham and Cheese (11g)

6" Roast Beef (12g)

6" Subway Club (12g)

6" Chicken Breast (10g)

6" Turkey Breast (10g)

Subway Club Salad (no dressing) (7g)

Taco Bell®

Taco (11g)

Chicken or Steak Soft Taco (10-11g)

Pintos and Cheese (9g)

Border Light Items (5-9g)

Mexican Rice (9g)

Wendy's®

Garden Salad (light dressing) (2g)

Junior Hamburger (9g)

Grilled Chicken (7g)

Small Chili (8g)

Baked Potato (2g)

Caesar Side Salad (5g)

Grilled Chicken Salad (8g)

Fat-free Dressing (0g)

When on Vacation

1. Know what you want to eat. Ask a native where they serve such foods.

2. Seek out a restaurant that:

   - Has plenty of low-fat options on the menu, including broiled fish, salad bar, fresh vegetables, stir-fried meals, or vegetable pizza, for example.

   - Does not exclusively serve high fat foods, such as French fries, hash brown potatoes, fried fish or chicken, or steaks.

   - Does not feature all-you-can-eat specials or buffets, as these promote overeating.

   - Will prepare food to order.

3. When traveling, bring an ice chest in the car filled with healthful foods: fresh fruits, cut-up raw vegetables, lean sandwich meats, low-fat cheese, low-fat crackers, bread, homemade potato or pasta salad, to name a few. Skim milk and cereal are easy breakfast foods.

4. Plan to stop along the roadside for breakfast and lunch to avoid overindulging at restaurants. But don't skip meals because this promotes overeating.

5. Special order airline food, with 24-hour notice.

Low-fat, Low Cholesterol, Low Triglyceride Diet

Limit cholesterol intake to 300 mg per day.
Consume no more than 25-35% of calories as fat.
Decrease alcohol and simple sugars.

Product	Recommended Servings	Choose	Avoid
Milk Products Milk	2-3 servings/day 1 cup = serving	Skim or 1% milkfat Non-fat dry milk solids, Skim evaporated milk, Skim buttermilk	2%, whole, chocolate milk Sweetened condensed milk Reg. evaporated milk Goat's milk – 48% fat
Cream		Poly Rich®, Non-fat dry milk powder, skim milk, Sour Cream Light or Fat-free Carnation®, Coffee-Mate Lite®, Fat-free Farm Ranch®	All kinds, such as Half & Half, Light, Heavy & Whipping Sour cream or imitation sour cream, Cool Whip® lite Non-dairy cream substitutes
Yogurt	1 cup (8 oz) = 1 serving	Skim or low-fat, Yogurt made with sugar substitute	Made from whole milk Low-fat frozen yogurt

Product	Recommended Servings	Choose	Avoid
Cottage Cheese	1/2 cup = serving	Low-fat or part skim milk with 5 gm. fat or less per ounce	Whole milk cheese with more than 5 grams per ounce Examples: cream cheese and Cheez Whiz
Cheese	1 1/2 - 2 oz. = serving 1 1/2 oz. natural cheese 2 oz. processed cheese	Examples: part skim mozzarella, Parmesan, Sap Sago®, Velveeta Light®, County Line Advantage® Individual slices: Borden's Lite-Line®, Kraft Lite 'N Lively® Loaf types, Cheezola®, Countdown®, Kraft Golden Image®, Healthy Favorites® Bulk types: Delicia®, Heidi Ann®, Kiss O' Swiss®, Kiss O' Gold®, Alpine Lace®, Hickory Farms® low cholesterol (bulk or cold pack)	Individual Slices: American cheese slices Loaf types: Velveeta®, Chef's Delight® Bulk types: Colby, longhorn, Swiss, County Line, Monterey Jack Fried Cheese

1,200 Calorie Menus
(Weight Loss Diet)

Note: This diet is based on women's calorie needs. For safe weight loss, men should add two starchy foods and one fruit daily for an extra 200 calories.

The average daily meal composition is 50% complex carbohydrates, 20% protein, and 30% fat.

The approximate calorie distributions are 25% for breakfast, 50% for lunch, and 25% for supper, as follows the 25-50-25 principle for optional weight loss.

IMPORTANT: This plan is low in calcium, in that it includes 300-500 milligrams of calcium a day (the recommended daily amount is 800 milligrams). As a result, if this diet is followed for more than 3 months, you should take a calcium supplement of 400-500 milligrams a day.

Days	Breakfast	Lunch	Dinner	Snack
Day 1	1/2 cup unsweetened orange juice (40) (c) 1 poached egg (80) (p) 1 slice whole wheat toast (70) (c) 1 tsp. tub margarine (35) (f) (total calories: 225)	1 cup vegetable soup (70) tuna sandwich: - 2 slices whole wheat bread (140) (c) - 1/2 cup water packed tuna (120) (p) - 1 tsp mayonnaise (35) (p) - lemon juice, pickle (f) 1 cup skim milk (80) (p, c) 1 small apple (50) (c) (total calories: 495)	2 oz broiled, skinless chicken (120) (p) 1 small baked potato (70) (c), with 1 tsp tub margarine (35) (f) 1/2 cup fresh carrots (20) (c) 1/2 cup fresh green beans (20) (c) 1 cup tossed lettuce/tomato/cucumber salad (20) (c) with herbed vinegar dressing (total calories: 285)	(Day's Total: 1,005)
Day 2	1/4 cantaloupe (45) (c), topped with 1/4 cup low-fat cottage cheese (50) (p) 1/2 whole wheat English muffin (70) (c) 1 tsp tub margarine (35) (f) 1/2 cup skim milk (40) (p, c) (total calories: 240)	turkey sandwich: - 2 slices whole wheat bread (140) (c); 2 oz turkey (120) (p); 1 tsp mayonnaise (35) (f); lettuce & tomato 1 small raw carrot, in sticks (20) (c) 1 medium pear (50) (c) Milk shake: 1 cup skim milk (80) (p,c); 1/4 banana (20) (c); 1 fresh peach or 2 unsweetened canned halves (40) (c), blended together (total calories: 505)	2 oz baked or broiled sole with lemon (110) (p) 1 small can of corn (70) (c) with 1 tsp tub margarine (35) (f) 1/2 cup steamed broccoli with lemon (20) (c) 1 cup tossed vegetable salad (20) (c), lemon vinegar dressing (total calories: 255)	(Day's Total: 1,000)

c=carbohydrates   f=fat   p=protein

125

Days	Breakfast	Lunch	Dinner	Snack
Day 3	1/2 small banana (40) (c) 3/4 cup dry whole wheat cereal, e.g., mini-shredded wheat (135) (c) 1 cup skim milk (80) (p, c) (total calories: 255)	1 cup lentil soup (165) (p, c) 1/2 cup low-fat cottage cheese (100) (p) atop 1 cup fresh fruit salad including citrus fruit (80) (c) 1 slice whole wheat toast (70) (c), with 1 tsp tub margarine (35) (f) 1 tomato, in wedges (20) (c) 1 cup spinach salad (30) (c), with herbal vinegar dressing (total calories: 500)	2 oz broiled veal chop (120) (p) 1/2 cup spaghetti (90) (c) 1 Tbsp Parmesan cheese (25) (p) 1/2 cup zucchini (8) (c) 1/2 cup cauliflower (12) (c) sliced cucumbers, with mint, dill, vinegar (total calories: 255)	(Day's Total: 1,010)
Day 4	1/2 grapefruit (40) (c) 1/2 cup hot oatmeal (75) (c), with cinnamon if desired and 1 tsp tub margarine (35) (f) 1 cup skim milk (80) (p, c) (total calories: 230)	2 oz roasted chicken (120) (p) 1/2 cup wild rice (110) (c) 1/2 cup green beans (20) (c) 1/2 cup carrot raisin salad: 1/2 cup shredded carrots (30) (c) 1 Tbsp raisins (20) (c) 1 tsp diet mayonnaise (15) (f) or 1 Tbsp unsweetened apple juice (15) (c) 1 small baked apple, with cinnamon (50) (c) (total calories: 380)	2 oz lean roast beef (120) (p) 1 small baked potato (70) (c) with 2 tsp diet margarine (30) (f) 1 cup yellow squash (15) (c) 1 cup tossed salad (20) (c), with 1 Tbsp herbed tomato juice dressing (total calories: 255)	1 nectarine (40) (c) (total calories: 40) (Day's Total: 905)

c=carbohydrates   f=fat   p=protein

Days	Breakfast	Lunch	Dinner	Snack
Day 5	cup fresh strawberries (40) (c) 1 slice whole wheat toast (70) (c) 1 Tbsp nonhydrogenated peanut butter (100) (p) 1/2 cup skim milk (40) (p, c) (total calories: 250)	1 cup tomato soup (75) (c) 1 "Cheese Pocket": 1 oz low-fat cheese, e.g., Mozzarella (80)(p), melted in 1 whole wheat pita (pocket) bread (140) (c) with lettuce, tomato, onion, mushrooms, and 1 tsp tub margarine (35) (f) relish tray and yogurt dip: 1 cup sliced cauliflower, broccoli, green pepper, celery, carrots, etc. (25) (c) 1/4 cup low-fat plain yogurt (40) (p, c) as dip, seasoned with 1/2 tsp dry onion flakes or 1/2 tsp ranch dressing mix 1 cup watermelon pieces (45) (c) 1 cup skim milk (80) (p, c) (total calories: 520)	2 oz broiled London broil (flank steak) (120) (p) 1/2 cup noodles (85) (c) cooked in chicken broth 1/2 cup carrots (20) (c) with parsley 1/2 cup steamed cabbage (20) (c), with lemon (total calories: 245)	**(Day's Total: 1,015)**
Day 6	1 cup unsweetened orange juice (40) (c) 1 whole wheat bagel (140) (c) 1 oz smoked turkey (60) (p) (total calories: 240)	1 hamburger: 1 whole wheat hamburger bun (140) (c) 2 oz lean ground beef (120) (p), mustard, lettuce, tomato, onion, pickle with 1 Tbsp mayo (35) (f) 1/2 cup ambrosia 1/2 cup mandarin orange and grapefruit sections) (40) (c), 1 Tbsp coconut & nuts (60) (f) 1 cup skim milk (80) (p, c) (total calories: 475)	seafood creole: 1 oz mixed seafood (110) (p), cooked in 1/2 cup tomato sauce with diced pepper, onion, celery (45)(c) 1/2 cup plain rice (80) (c) 1/2 cup tossed salad (20) (c) 1 Tbsp herbed vinegar dressing (total calories: 255)	1 medium peach (40) (c) (total calories: 40) **(Day's Total: 1,010)**

c=carbohydrates   f=fat   p=protein

Days	Breakfast	Lunch	Dinner	Snack
Day 7	1 small banana (80) (c) 1 cheese toast: 1 oz low-fat cheese (e.g., farmer's cheese) (80) (p) melted 1 slice whole wheat bread (70) (c) 1/2 cup skim milk (40) (p, c)	Chinese stir-fry dinner: 2 oz sliced chicken (120) (p), and 1 cup mixed vegetables: sliced broccoli, mushrooms, onions, snowpeas, celery, carrots, bamboo shoots, water chestnuts, almonds (45) (c), cooked in 2 tsp oil (70) (f), 2 tsp soy sauce 1/2 cup brown rice (90) (c) 1 cup tossed salad (20) (c) with 1 Tbsp low-calorie dressing (20) (f) Hawaiian salad: 3/4 cup strawberries, banana, pineapple (60) (c) 1/2 cup skim milk (40) (p, c)	stuffed tomato: 1 tomato (20) (c), filled with 1/2 cup water packed tuna or salmon (120) (p), 1 tsp mayonnaise (35) (f), diced green pepper, celery, onion, parsley, seasonings 1/2 cup cucumber, sliced 4 whole wheat crackers (55) (c)	2 small or 1 medium plum (45)
	(total calories: 270)	(total calories: 465)	(total calories: 230)	(total calories: 45) **(Day's Total: 1,010)**

c=carbohydrates   f=fat   p=protein

Other Healthy Menu Suggestions

Days	Breakfast	Lunch	Dinner	Snacks	Notes
Monday	6 oz orange juice 2 shredded wheat biscuits with skim milk, 2 slices whole wheat toast 1 Tbsp jam, decaf hot beverage	grilled fat-free cheese sandwich whole wheat bread, 1/2 cup low-fat cottage cheese, 1 cup low-fat chicken noodle soup, 8 fat-free saltines, 1 diet caffeine free drink	tossed salad with 4 tsp fat-free dressing, baked skinless chicken breast, 1 med baked potato with fat-free sour cream or dressing, 1 cup green beans, 1 cup fruit cocktail, decaffeinated coffee or tea	10 a.m. med apple or 7 in banana

2 p.m. low-fat Twinkie®

8 p.m. 1 cup fat-free yogurt with fat-free chocolate sauce | |
| Tuesday | 6 oz apple juice, 3 oz dry oatmeal 1/2 cup skim milk, 1 slice whole wheat toast with 1 tsp jam, decaf | Lettuce and tomato salad with 4 tsp fat free dressing, 3 oz tuna sandwich, 2 tsp fat-free mayo, 2 slices whole wheat bread, 6 oz carton fat-free yogurt, low-fat cupcake, 1 diet caffeine free drink | Raw carrots with fat-free ranch, baked skinless chicken breast, 1 cup mashed potatoes use skim milk fat free margarine, 1 cup lima beans, 1 small whole wheat dinner roll, 8 oz skim milk | 10 a.m. 3 double fat-free graham crackers

2 p.m. 1 sliced apple with low-fat caramel sauce

8 p.m. slice angel food cake | |

Days	Breakfast	Lunch	Dinner	Snacks	Notes
Wednesday	6 oz grapefruit juice, egg beater omelet onion, green pepper, mushrooms, 1 slice fat-free cheese, 1 slice Canadian bacon, 1 English muffin, decaffeinated beverage	2 slices whole wheat bread with 2 slices fat free cheese and fat-free condiment, 1 cup tomato soup, 1/2 cup applesauce with 3 low-fat vanilla wafers, 1 caffeine-free diet drink	Tossed salad with 4 tsp fat-free dressing, 3 oz baked fish, baked potato with fat-free sour cream or dressing, 1 cup broccoli; 1/2 a canned peach with 1/2 cup fat-free pudding, caffeine-free diet drink	10 a.m. low-fat uncoated granola bar 2 p.m. 2 rice cakes 8 p.m. 1/2 cup Grape-Nuts® 1 oz skim milk 1 packet sweetener	
Thursday	6 oz choice juice, 1 cup rice krispies with 1/2 cup skim milk, 1 banana, 1 slice whole wheat toast with Tbsp peanut butter, decaf beverage	1 veggie burger on 2 slices whole wheat bread may add free veggies and tsp fat-free condiment, 1/2 cup baked beans, 6 oz yogurt cup, 1 apple or orange, decaffeinated drink	Lettuce salad with fat-free dressing, 1 cup spaghetti with 1/2 cup marinara sauce, 1 plain bread stick, 1/2 cup low-fat ice cream, decaf beverage	10 a.m. choice of fruit 2 p.m. low-fat granola bar 8 p.m. low-fat cupcake, Twinkie, or brownie	

Days	Breakfast	Lunch	Dinner	Snacks	Notes
Friday	2 - 6" pancakes with fat-free sugar- free syrup, 1 low- fat smokey link, 6 oz skim milk, decaffeinated beverage	1 McDonald's® plain hamburger, 1 medium apple, low-fat cupcake, caffeine-free diet drink	1/2 cup low-fat cottage cheese, 1/2 cup peach slices, 3 oz hamburger steak broiled, 1 cup cooked carrots, 1 slice angel food cake with 2 tsp strawberry topping, caffeine-free diet beverage	10 a.m. choice of fruit 2 p.m. 12 small fat-free pretzels 8 p.m. 1 toasted English muffin with jam	
Saturday					
Sunday					

Your Personal Menu Chart

Days	Breakfast	Lunch	Dinner	Snacks	Notes
Monday					
Tuesday					

Days	Breakfast	Lunch	Dinner	Snacks	Notes
Wednesday					
Thursday					

Days	Breakfast	Lunch	Dinner	Snacks	Notes
Friday					
Saturday					

134

Healthy Eating Book List

Making Healthy Choices away from Home

Florman, Monte, and Marjorie Florman. *Fast Foods: Eating in and Eating Out.* Consumers Union, 1990.

Franz, Marion J. *Fast Food Fasts: Nutrition and Exchange Values for Fast-Food Restaurants*, 3rd ed. DCI Publishers, 1990.

Kanersloot, Mary. *The Fast Food Diet: Quick and Healthy Eating at Home and on the Go.* Simon & Schuster, 1991.

Warshaw, Hope S. *The Restaurant Companion: A Guide to Healthier Eating Out.* Surrey Books, 1990.

Selected Cookbooks for Healthy Eating

Brody, Jane. *Good Food Book: Living the High Carbohydrate Way.* Norton, New York Publishers, 1985.

Cone, Marcia, and Thelma Snyder. *Microwave Diet Cookery.* Simon & Schuster, 1998.

Cooking Light, Cookbook Series. Oxmoor House, 1991.

Cooper, Nancy. *The Joy of Snacks.* Diabetes Center, 1991.

Gilliard, Judy, and Joy Kirkpatrick. *The Guiltless Gourmet Goes Ethnic: Low in Fat, Cholesterol, Salt, Sugar, Calories.* DCI Publishing, 1990.

Harsil, Janis, and Evie Hansen. *Light-Hearted Seafood.* National Seafood Educators, 1989.

The Healthy Holiday Cookbook. American Heart Association, Iowa Affiliate, 1988.

Hinman, Bobbie, and Millie Snyder. *More Lean and Luscious by Bobbie Hinman and Millie Snyder.* Prima Pub. & Communications/St. Martin's Press, 1988.

Landholz, Edna, et. al. *Over 50 and Still Cooking: Recipes for Good Health and Long Life*. Bristol Publishers, 1990.

Lindsay, Anne. *The American Cancer Society Cookbook: A Menu for Good Health*. Hearst Books, 1988.

Miller, Jeannette, and Carol Van Waardhuizen. *The Healthy Holiday Cookbook*, 2nd ed. American Heart Association, Iowa Affiliate, 1988.

Ponichter, Brenda J. *Quick and Healthy*. 1991.

Smith, M.J. *All-American Low-Fat Meals in Minutes: Recipes and Menus for Special Occasions or Every Day*. DCI Publishing, 1990.

Starke, Rodman D., and Mary Winston, ed. *American Heart Association Low-Salt Cookbook: A Complete Guide to Reducing Sodium and Fat in the Diet*. Times Books, 1990.

Williams, Lucy M. *Recipes for the Heart: A Nutrition Guide for People with High Blood Pressure*. Sandridge Publishers, 1988.

Sports Nutrition

Clark, Nancy. *Nancy Clark's Sports Nutrition Guidebook*. Leisure Press, 1990.

Coleman, Ellen. *Eating for Endurance*. Bull Publishing Co., 1988.

Peterson, Marilyn S., and Keith Peterson. *Eat to Compete: A Guide to Sports Nutrition*. Year Book Medical Publishers, 1988.

Smith, Nathan J., and Bonnie Worthington-Roberts. *Food for Sport*. Bull Publishing Co., 1989.

On Reducing Fat and Cholesterol

American Heart Association. *Low-Fat, Low-Cholesterol Cookbook*. Random House, 1989.

Anderson, James W. *Be Heart Smart...The HCF Way to a Healthy Heart.* HCF Nutrition Research Foundation, Inc., 1989.

Connor, Sonja L., and William E. Connor. *The New American Diet System.* Simon and Schuster, 1991.

Consumer Guide, ed. *Cholesterol: Your Guide for a Healthy Heart.* Publications International, 1989.

Cooper, Kenneth. *Controlling Cholesterol.* Bantam Books, 1988.

Fletcher, Anne M. *Eat Fish, Live Better.* Harper & Row, 1989.

Goor, Ron, and Nancy Goor. *Eater's Choice: A Food Lover's Guide to Lower Cholesterol.* Houghton Mifflin, 1989.

Griffen, Glen O., and William P. Castelli. *Good Fat, Bad Fat: How to Lower Your Cholesterol and Beat the Odds of a Heart Attack.* Fisher Books, 1989.

Hachfeld, Linda, and Betsy Eykryn. *Cooking a la Heart.* Appletree Press, 1991

Kwiterovich, Peter. *Beyond Cholesterol.* John Hopkins University Press, 1989.

Lindsay, Anne. *Low Cholesterol Cuisine.* Hearst Books, 1989.

Ornish, Dean. *Dr. Dean Ornish's Program for Reversing Heart Disease: The Only System Scientifically Proven to Reverse Heart Disease without Drugs or Surgery.* Random House, 1990.

Piscatella, Jo. *Controlling Your Fat Tooth.* 1991.

Smith, M.J., MA, RD, LD. *All-American Low-Fat Meals in Minutes.* John Wiley & Sons, Inc., 1990.

Ulene, Art, ed. *Count Out Cholesterol Cookbook: A Feeling Fine Book.* A. A. Knopf, 1989.

Wilson, Nedra P., and Susan M. Wood. *Delicious Ways to Lower Cholesterol.* Oxmoor House, Inc., 1989.

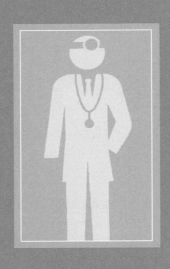

CHAPTER SEVEN

Working with Medical Professionals

We have talked a great deal about the fast-paced world in which we live today and how important it is to develop a healthy lifestyle for ultimate wellness.

As we maintain our health, it is important to maintain regular contact with medical professionals as well. It is also important to know how to prepare for an appointment with the doctor, including what information to share and what questions to ask.

This chapter offers information about how you can work and interact productively and successfully with health care givers.

Health Screening

As the body ages checkups become even more important to detect potential health problems. The following chart shows the recommended routine screenings for adults.

Test or Procedure	Who Needs It	How Often
Blood pressure measurement	All adults	Every two years for those with normal blood pressure; more for those with readings of 130/85 or higher.
Cholesterol measurement	All adults	Once every 5 years; more often if LDL ("bad") is high or HDL ("good") is low.
Pap Smear	All women starting at age 20 or when sexually active	If three annual tests are normal then once every three years based on your risk factors and as recommended by your doctor.
Mammogram (breast X-ray)	Baseline at age 35-39 with risk factors; Women ages 40-49; Women ages 50 and over	Based on doctor's recommendations after assessing risk factors.
Yearly Prostate screening: DRE (digital rectal exam), PSA (prostate specific antigen)	Men with family history; starting at age 40 for DRE and PSA. For other men, starting at age 50 for DRE and possible PSA	DRE annually PSA on professional advice
Rubella vaccine	All women of childbearing age	Once

Test or Procedure	Who Needs It	How Often
Colon cancer	Everyone age 50 and older/ earlier for those at risk	• Flexible sigmoidoscopy, every 2-3 years after age 50 • Colon X-ray every 2 years with high risks or every 4 years if not high risk after age 50 • Colonoscopy every 10 years after age 50 if not at high risk; every 2 years if high risk, or every 6 months if at risk
Glucose (for diabetes)	Everyone age 45 and older/ earlier for those at risk	Once a year
Glaucoma screening	People at high risk/those over age 65/very near-sighted or diabetic	On professional advice of eye specialist
Tetanus/diphtheria booster	All adults	Every 10 years or after a deep or dirty wound if most recent shot was more than 5 years ago
Hepatitis A	Travelers and people in high risk groups (chronic liver disease or people who have had contact with some-one who has had hepatitis A)	On professional advice
Hepatitis B	Health care workers as well as adults at high risk	On professional advice
Dental checkup	All adults	Every 6 months on professional advice
Thyroid disease	Women age 50 and over	On professional advice

Health History

Name: _____

Street Address: _____

City, State, Zip: _____

Phone: _____

Date of Birth: _____

Blood Type: _____

Emergency Contact #1: _____

(Relationship) _____

Street Address: _____

City, State, Zip: _____

Phone: _____

Emergency Contact #2: _____

(Relationship) _____

Street Address: _____

City, State, Zip: _____

Phone: _____

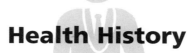

Health History

Current Prescription Medications:

_____

_____

_____

_____

_____

_____

_____

_____

_____

_____

Current Over-the-Counter Medications:

_____

_____

_____

_____

_____

_____

_____

_____

Health History

Allergies/Sensitivities:

_____

_____

_____

_____

_____

_____

Surgeries: (date, procedure, length of hospital stay)

_____

_____

_____

_____

_____

Other Hospitalizations (date, reason, length)

_____

_____

_____

_____

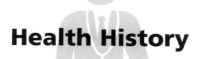

Health History

Minor Surgeries (Screenings/treatments with dates completed)

_____

_____

_____

_____

_____

_____

Insurance: (list **all** with policy numbers)

_____

_____

_____

_____

_____

Primary Physician: (or medical provider)

_____

Specialty: _____

Address: _____

Phone: _____

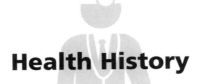

Health History

Other Medical Provider: _____

Specialty: _____

Address: _____

Phone: _____

_____

Other Medical Provider: _____

Specialty: _____

Address: _____

Phone: _____

_____

Other Medical Provider: _____

Specialty: _____

Address: _____

Phone: _____

_____

Other Screening Information: _____

_____

_____

_____

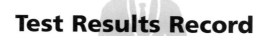

Test Results Record

Test_____ Date_____

Reason:_____

Result:_____

_____

Follow-up:_____

Test_____ Date_____

Reason:_____

Result:_____

_____

Follow-up:_____

Test_____ Date_____

Reason:_____

Result:_____

_____

Follow-up:_____

Immunization Record

Vaccine	Date	Place
Tetanus Diphtheria (Td) (booster every 10 years)		
Pneumonia At least once (65 years of age or older)		
Flu Every year after 50		

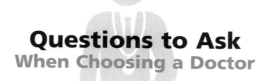

Questions to Ask
When Choosing a Doctor

What are the doctor's professional qualifications:

- License to practice
- Certification by medical specialty board
- Hospital affiliation

What is the doctor's and/or office accessibility:

- Does he/she have a call-in hour for you to ask questions?
- Will he/she refer you to other specialists when needed?
- Will he/she care for you if you are hospitalized?

Communication:

- Does he/she offer you an opportunity to ask questions?
- Does he/she respond in an open and understandable way?
- Does he/she discuss with you the proposed treatment of your illness?
- Does he/she encourage your cooperation in treatment?

Practice Environment:

Your physician and his or her staff should treat you with respect and courtesy. Considerate treatment includes:

- A minimal amount of waiting time
- A clean, fresh office
- Confidential handling of health information
- Privacy during interviews, examinations, treatments, and consultations
- Willingness to discuss and explain fees and billing practices
- Help in completing routine insurance forms, if requested

Preparations for a Doctor's Visit

To prepare for a visit with your doctor:

- Make a list of all of your questions.
- Make a list of all of your medications.
- Talk over your concerns with your doctor. Never withhold information from your doctor.
- State the reason for your visit.
- State as clearly as you can the changes in body functions, from sleep and bowel habits to other changes such as headaches.

Questions to ask at the visit:

- What is wrong with me?
- What treatments are available?
- Which treatment do you recommend? Why do you recommend this treatment?
- Are there any risks with this treatment?
- What medicines are you going to prescribe? What are they for?
- Will I feel any differently during the treatment?
- What are the side effects of treatment and/or medication? What should I do if I experience any of them?
- When will there be an improvement in my condition?
- Would I benefit from seeing a specialist?

In evaluating your physician, the ultimate consideration is your personal satisfaction with the medical care you receive. Do you feel you have a comfortable relationship with your physician? Do you trust and have confidence in his or her ability to provide you with high quality medical care?

Eight reasons to leave your doctor . . .

1. Poor bedside manner

2. Too vague and evasive

3. Never on schedule

4. Can't diagnose the problem

5. Orders too many tests

6. Discourages second opinions

7. Doesn't protect medical privacy

8. Unpleasant office staff

Questions to Ask
Your Doctor When the Diagnosis Is Serious

- What kind of _____ do I have?
- How far has this progressed? What does this mean?
- If it hasn't progressed, how long before it progresses or progresses further?
- Are more tests needed? If so, what are they?
- When and where will the tests be done?
- How long will each test take?
- What are the risks and benefits associated with each test?
- Do I need to bring someone with me to the test?
- What are my treatment options?
- What is the recommended treatment?
- What are the side effects?
- Will I get ill?
- What are the long-term and short-term results?
- What is my projected quality of life during and after treatment?
- Will I have to quit working?
- What can I do to help myself (diet, exercise, vitamins)?
- Is there a support group or other available information?

Take a relative or friend with you for the appointment. You can also take a note pad or tape recorder to record the information so that after the meeting you can discuss the information and review your options.

Questions to Ask
Your Surgeon Before the Surgery

When meeting with your physician and/or surgeon before a surgery, consider asking these questions.

- What operation are you recommending?
- Why do I need this operation?
- What do you expect the surgery to achieve?
- Could you please explain the entire procedure?
- How many times have you performed this operation?
- What will happen if I don't have the surgery?
- Should I get a second opinion?
- What are the risks involved in the surgery?
- How do the benefits outweigh the risks?
- What tests will I need to have before surgery?
- Is there anything else that will need to be done before surgery?
- What kind of anesthesia will I need?
- How long will I have to be in the hospital?
- How will I feel after the surgery?
- How will my pain be controlled?
- What symptoms should be reported to you after the surgery?
- Will the surgery have any negative long-term effects?
- How long will it be before I can go home?

- Will any rehabilitation be needed?
- Will any other physicians be caring for me? If so, who are they and how were they selected?
- How long before I can resume my normal activities?
- Will the cost be covered by my insurance?

Take a relative or friend with you for the interview. After the meeting you can discuss the information with him/her and review your options.

Questions to Ask
Your Pharmacist

When filling a prescription, ask your pharmacist for information.

- What are the generic and trade names of this drug?
- What is the medication for?
- Can a generic drug be substituted?
- How long will it take this medicine to work?
- What will happen if I do not take this medicine?
- Should I keep taking the medicine until the prescription is gone or until the symptoms are gone?
- What should I do if I miss a dose?
- Do I take this drug with food?
- Should I avoid any types of food, beverage, or other medicines while I am taking this drug?
- Should alcohol be avoided while taking this drug?
- Will smoking affect the way this drug works?
- While taking this drug should I avoid any activities (driving, exercise, sun exposure)?
- What side effects can I expect from this medication? Which ones should I report to the doctor?
- How should I store this medication?
- Can I get this prescription refilled?
- Can I get a larger quantity of the medication so it will last longer and cost less?

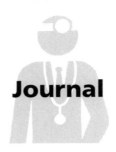

Journal

As part of living a healthy life, it is very important that the adult caregiver in the family maintains the medical records for the family. Use this journal as a tool to keep track of what is happening with you and your family. Things to record include: tests; procedures; breathing exercises; schedule of doctor, nurse, or therapist visits; medications and medication times.

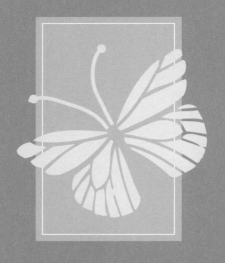

CHAPTER 8

Wellness Tools

There are many tools available for use as we make our individual plans to be able to "be well to serve well." In this chapter you will find wellness resources that should be beneficial in organizing and planning a wellness program for individuals and groups.

These tried-and-true guides can be programmed to fit your personalized needs. Choose those that best fit your assessed needs and get underway, so you and your family may enjoy life to its fullest.

A DAY PLANNED: A Tool

5:30 a.m. Sweet, beautiful music breaks into the beautiful dream. This is a new time the Lord has given. Let us rejoice and be glad!

CAREGIVERS

- ☐ 5:30-6:00 a.m. Time with God
- ☐ 6:00-6:45 a.m. Get ready for the day
- ☐ 6:45-7:30 a.m. Get the family up for breakfast
- ☐ Ready for Work-School-Chores-Travel for the day

SCHEDULE TIME FOR YOUR FAMILY AND YOU

- ☐ 8:00-9:00 a.m.
- ☐ 9:00-10:00 a.m
- ☐ 10:00-11:00 a.m.
- ☐ 11:00 a.m.-Noon
- ☐ 12:00-1:00 p.m.
- ☐ 1:00-2:00 p.m.
- ☐ 2:00-3:00 p.m.

- ☐ 3:00-4:00 p.m.
- ☐ 4:00-5:00 p.m.
- ☐ 5:00-6:00 p.m.
- ☐ 6:00-7:00 p.m.
- ☐ 7:00-8:00 p.m.
- ☐ 8:00-9:00 p.m.
- ☐ Bed

DAILY WORKOUT: Level One
4 times per week (for 3 weeks)

WARM UP 3 MINUTES TO TIME

☐ 20 jumping jacks

☐ 20 deep knee bends

☐ 10 left side stretches

☐ 10 right side stretches

☐ 10 middle stretches

☐ 30 abdominal crunches
(with 5 second rest between each set of 10)

☐ 30 abdominal crunches with knee crossed to left
(with 5 second rest between each set of 10)

☐ 30 Abdominal crunches with knee crossed to right
(with 5 second rest between each set of 10)

☐ 30 sit ups *(with 5 second rest between each set of 10)*

☐ 30 abdominal crunches *(with both legs lifted 3 inches)*
(with 5 second rest between each set of 10)

☐ 30 minutes walking *(15-minute mile)*

DAILY WORKOUT: Level Two
4 times per week (for 3 weeks)

WARM UP 3 MINUTES TO TIME

☐ 20 jumping jacks

☐ 20 deep knee bends

☐ 10 left side stretches

☐ 10 right side stretches

☐ 10 middle stretches

☐ 50 abdominal crunches *(with 5 second rest between each set of 50)*

☐ 50 abdominal crunches with knee crossed to left
(with 5 second rest between each set of 50)

☐ 50 abdominal crunches with knee crossed to right
(with 5 second rest between each set of 50)

☐ 50 sit ups with 5 lb. weight on stomach*
(with 5 second rest between each set of 50)

☐ 50 abdominal crunches with 1 lb. weight on ankles*
(with both legs lifted 3 inches, and 5 second rest between each set of 50)

☐ 50 inside thigh lifts *(with 5 second rest between each set of 50)*

☐ 50 outside thigh lifts *(with 5 second rest between each set of 50)*

☐ 40 minutes run/walk *(2 minutes run, 2 minutes walk)*

*You can use canned vegetables or household items for weights

DAILY WORKOUT: Level Three
4 times per week (for life)

WARM UP 3 MINUTES TO TIME

- [ ] 20 jumping jacks
- [ ] 20 deep knee bends
- [ ] 10 left side stretches
- [ ] 10 right side stretches
- [ ] 10 middle stretches
- [ ] 100 abdominal crunches *(with 5 second rest between each set of 100)*
- [ ] 100 abdominal crunches with knee crossed to left *(with 5 second rest between each set of 100)*
- [ ] 100 abdominal crunches with knee crossed to right *(with 5 second rest between each set of 100)*
- [ ] 100 sit ups with 10 lb. weight on stomach* *(with 5 second rest between each set of 100)*
- [ ] 100 abdominal crunches with 2 lb. weight on ankles* *(with both legs lifted 3 inches, and 5 second rest between each set of 100)*
- [ ] 100 inside thigh lifts *(with 5 second rest between each set of 100)*
- [ ] 100 outside thigh lifts *(with 5 second rest between each set of 100)*
- [ ] 60 minutes cardiovscular exercise: walk 4 miles *(15 minutes or less each mile)*

*You can use canned vegetables or household items for weights

Principles of a Low-fat, Low Cholesterol Lifestyle

These principles of a low-fat, low cholesterol diet are essential for a healthy lifestyle because:

- A diet low in saturated fat helps to prevent coronary artery disease.

- A diet low in total fat lowers the risk of developing cancer and promotes weight loss or maintenance of a healthy weight.

- A diet rich in fruits and vegetables helps to lower the risk of cancer and heart disease due to the fiber, vitamin C, and other natural substances they contain.

- Consumption of sugar promotes tooth decay but poses no other risk (for non-diabetics) when consumed in a well-balanced meal plan.

- Fiber from complex carbohydrates (grain products) tends to lower cholesterol and reduces the risk of colon cancer.

- Sodium intake should be controlled in the case of high blood pressure, congestive heart failure, or problems with retaining fluid. A moderate sodium limit is recommended for otherwise healthy individuals.

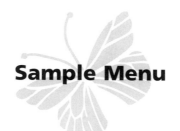

Sample Menu

BREAKFAST
Shredded Wheat
Orange Juice
Whole Wheat Toast (with jelly)
Egg Beaters
Skim Milk (1 cup)
Decaffeinated Coffee

LUNCH
Toasted Cheese Sandwich
    (use Kraft Free or Healthy Choice cheese
    and butter flavored cooking spray to grill)
Green Beans
Lettuce Salad (with 1 Tbsp. French dressing)
Fruit
Graham Crackers
Skim Milk (1 cup)

DINNER
Baked Chicken (without skin)
Mashed Potatoes
Broccoli
Sliced Tomatoes
Whole Wheat Bread (with jelly)
Gelatin
Decaffeinated Coffee

Ten Terrific Resolutions

Slip gently into a healthier way of living, without starving yourself or running yourself ragged. Sticking with just one of these resolutions will put you well on the road to looking and feeling better.

Resolution #1: "I will watch fat not calories."

Excess fat is the number one dietary villain. A good goal for most adults is to limit "fat calories" to 30 percent of total calories. That's up to 667 "calories from fat" for women eating 2,000 calories per day and 833 "calories from fat" for men taking in 2,500 calories. Thanks to nutrition labels, keeping track of fat is fairly easy. Even some fast-food restaurants offer nutrition information.

Resolution #2: "I will heed the 3 gram rule."

Foods that have more than 3 grams of fat per 100 calories should be balanced with low-fat foods. So if you opt for a 600 calorie frozen dinner with 30 grams of fat, augment it with an unbuttered vegetable or bread and fresh fruit for dessert.

Resolution #3: "I will make a menu."

Planning your meals once a week reduces the "what's-for-dinner" stress, while it almost guarantees healthful eating. Take a "backward" approach. Start your menus with vegetables, fruits, and grain products (bread, rice, pasta). Then add two-to four-ounce servings of poultry, fish, and cheese.

Don't forget to plan for restaurant meals and take-along lunches. Take along your menu and concentrate on salads and broiled selections.

Resolution #4: "I will fill up on flavor and fiber."

Fat in food adds flavor and leaves you feeling satisfied when you're done eating. Fortunately, there are ways to achieve these same benefits without the penalties that come with fat. To add flavor, stock up on spices, herbs, flavored vinegars, and condiments like soy sauce and Dijon mustard. Experiment with new flavorings on a regular basis. Don't forget that herbs and spices lose their vigor after a while, so throw away the old supply and buy small amounts as you need them.

To create that "push-back-from-the-table" feeling of fullness, increase the amount of fiber in your meals. Grains, fruits, and vegetables are excellent sources of fill-you-up fiber and are low in fat, provided you don't slather on butter or drown them in fatty sauces. Another tip: An 8 ounce glass of water with your meals helps fill you up and improve digestion.

Resolution #5: "I will reform my shopping list."

The food you put in your shopping cart is the food that winds up on your plate (and hips). Load up on quality, healthful foods, and good eating will follow. Fruits, vegetables, breads, and seafood are excellent and tasty additions to any food basket. But as you make up your weekly list (right after you create your menu), try the following switches:

For:	Substitute:
Whole milk	Skim milk
High-fat cheeses (cheddar, blue, etc.)	Lower-fat cheeses (mozzarella, feta, etc.)
Rib eye steak	Round, sirloin, flank
Snack chips	Pretzels, plain popcorn
Frozen fried chicken dinner	Frozen baked cod dinner
Luncheon meats	Extra lean ham, Canadian bacon
Ice cream	Frozen yogurt
Chocolate chip cookies	Fig bars, gingersnaps
Yellow cake mix	Angel food cake mix
Breakfast Danish	Raisin bagel
Ground chuck	Ground round
Pepperoni pizza	Mushroom pizza

Resolution #6: "I will deliver myself from temptation."

Most "sinful" foods can fit into a healthful diet, provided you eat them in modest proportions. No one ever got fat eating half a cup of ice cream once a week. And 1/12 of a chocolate cake isn't going to do near the damage as half the cake.

Of course, not all of us are saintly enough to withstand temptation. So banish your downfall foods from home. Then make a monthly or weekly pilgrimage to your local temple of sweets, vowing beforehand to limit yourself.

Resolution #7: "I will activate my lifestyle."

Your diet probably isn't what is adding those extra pounds, says obesity expert Kelly Brownell, Ph.D. As proof, he notes that the average American eats about the same number of calories today as in the 1930s; at that time the average person worked off about 2,600 calories daily beyond what is needed to keep our body warm and functioning. Today we burn only about 600 activity calories each day.

There are lots of ways to bring your activity levels more in line with your calorie intake. Jogging and walking are two excellent, efficient ways. Dr. Brownell suggests that we simply get back into the habit of "doing" things.

Five examples:

- Take the stairs.
- Park as far as you can from the door.
- Push a lawn mower.
- Wash and dry the dishes yourself.
- Hide the remote control.

Resolution #8: "I will start a walking program."

Walking is the one exercise that almost every health expert can agree on. It is easy on your body, requires no special skills or equipment, and can be enjoyed by anyone in reasonably good shape. (Still, check with your doctor before starting any exercise if you are over 35 years of age or have medical problems.)

A surprisingly small amount of walking can reap big results. Studies by Ralph Paffenberger, M.D., indicate that burning about 300 calories in activity each day can add years to your life and add life to your years. To burn 300 or so calories, you would need to walk about 3 miles — that is 45-60 minutes for most people. But if you've pledged yourself to Resolution #7, you will need somewhat less formal exercise to reach your 300 calorie goal. Here is how to get started:

- Use the car odometer, drive a half mile from home in several directions.

- Each day pick one route and walk it out and back. Don't hurry.

- When you can comfortably walk each route in 15 minutes, increase your distance to 2 miles round-trip.

- Increase to 3 miles when you can cover 2 miles in 30 minutes.

- Your final goal is 3 miles in 45 minutes. Beginners, expect to spend 8-12 weeks reaching this goal.

Resolution #9: "I will bag a buddy."

Exercisers who walk or work out with a partner are much more likely to keep at it, according to several studies. Whether it is the camaraderie or the peer pressure, no one is certain why the buddy system seems to work. Clearly, though, pairing up with a friend or spouse is the best move you can make when starting an exercise program.

Resolution #10: "I will ride a bike, not a bandwagon."

A lot of people seem to think of healthful eating and regular exercise as bandwagons they would like to jump on. Unfortunately, when you fall off a bandwagon, it continues to roll on, out of reach. "This is true for smoking. Remember to keep on trying and you will eventually stay on the bike," says Paul R. Kipp, M.D.

You will do much better if you think of these resolutions as bicycles. If you fall off, so what? It is not a problem to climb back on, and you have learned something to boot. So no matter how often you fall off, don't lose heart. The more often you try, the better you will get. And, like bike riding, once your body learns how to live more healthfully, it will never forget.

Reprinted from *Better Homes and Gardens*, January 1991

Height & Weight Chart
for Women

Frame Size

Height Ft. In.	Small	Medium	Large
4'10"	102-111	109-121	118-131
4'11"	103-113	111-123	120-134
5'0"	104-115	113-126	122-137
5'1"	106-118	115-129	125-140
5'2"	108-121	118-132	128-143
5'3"	111-124	121-135	131-147
5'4"	114-127	124-138	134-151
5'5"	117-130	127-141	137-155
5'6"	120-133	130-144	140-159
5'7"	123-136	133-144	143-163
5'8"	126-139	136-150	146-167
5'9"	129-142	139-153	149-170
5'10"	132-145	142-156	152-173
5'11"	135-148	145-159	155-176
6'0"	138-151	148-162	158-176

Height & Weight Chart
for Men

Frame Size

Height Ft. In.	Small	Medium	Large
5'2"	128-134	131-141	138-150
5'3"	130-136	133-143	140-153
5'4"	132-138	135-145	142-156
5'5"	134-140	137-148	144-160
5'6"	136-142	139-151	146-164
5'7"	138-145	142-154	149-168
5'8"	140-148	145-157	152-172
5'9"	142-151	156-160	155-176
5'10"	144-154	151-163	158-180
5'11"	146-157	154-166	161-184
6'0"	149-160	157-170	164-188
6'1"	152-164	160-174	168-192
6'2"	155-168	165-178	172-197
6'3"	158-172	167-182	176-202
6'4"	162-176	171-187	181-207

Normal = BMI 19–24 **Overweight** = BMI 25–29 **Obese** = BMI 30–39 **Extreme Obesity** = BMI 40–54

Body Weight (pounds)

Height (inches) \ BMI	19	20	21	22	23	24	25	26	27	28	29	30	31	32	33	34	35	36	37	38	39	40	41	42	43	44	45	46	47	48	49	50	51	52	53	54
58	91	96	100	105	110	115	119	124	129	134	138	143	148	153	158	162	167	172	177	181	186	191	196	201	205	210	215	220	224	229	234	239	244	248	253	258
59	94	99	104	109	114	119	124	128	133	138	143	148	153	158	163	168	173	178	183	188	193	198	203	208	212	217	222	227	232	237	242	247	252	257	262	267
60	97	102	107	112	118	123	128	133	138	143	148	153	158	163	168	174	179	184	189	194	199	204	209	215	220	225	230	235	240	245	250	255	261	266	271	276
61	100	106	111	116	122	127	132	137	143	148	153	158	164	169	175	180	185	190	195	201	206	211	217	222	227	232	238	243	248	254	259	264	269	275	280	285
62	104	109	115	120	126	131	136	142	147	153	158	164	169	175	180	186	191	196	202	207	213	218	224	229	235	240	246	251	256	262	267	273	278	284	289	295
63	107	113	118	124	130	135	141	146	152	158	163	169	175	180	186	191	197	203	208	214	220	225	231	237	242	248	254	259	265	270	278	282	287	293	299	304
64	110	116	122	128	134	140	145	151	157	163	169	174	180	186	192	197	204	209	215	221	227	232	238	244	250	256	262	267	273	279	285	291	296	302	308	314
65	114	120	126	132	138	144	150	156	162	168	174	180	186	192	198	204	210	216	222	228	234	240	246	252	258	264	270	276	282	288	294	300	306	312	318	324
66	118	124	130	136	142	148	155	161	167	173	179	186	192	198	204	210	216	223	229	235	241	247	253	260	266	272	278	284	291	297	303	309	315	322	328	334
67	121	127	134	140	146	153	159	166	172	178	185	191	198	204	211	217	223	230	236	242	249	255	261	268	274	280	287	293	299	306	312	319	325	331	338	344
68	125	131	138	144	151	158	164	171	177	184	190	197	203	210	216	223	230	236	243	249	256	262	269	276	282	289	295	302	308	315	322	328	335	341	348	354
69	128	135	142	149	155	162	169	176	182	189	196	203	209	216	223	230	236	243	250	257	263	270	277	284	291	297	304	311	318	324	331	338	345	351	358	365
70	132	139	146	153	160	167	174	181	188	195	202	209	216	222	229	236	243	250	257	264	271	278	285	292	299	306	313	320	327	334	341	348	355	362	369	376
71	136	143	150	157	165	172	179	186	193	200	208	215	222	229	236	243	250	257	265	272	279	286	293	301	308	315	322	329	338	343	351	358	365	372	379	386
72	140	147	154	162	169	177	184	191	199	206	213	221	228	235	242	250	258	265	272	279	287	294	302	309	316	324	331	338	346	353	361	368	375	383	390	397
73	144	151	159	166	174	182	189	197	204	212	219	227	235	242	250	257	265	272	280	288	295	302	310	318	325	333	340	348	355	363	371	378	386	393	401	408
74	148	155	163	171	179	186	194	202	210	218	225	233	241	249	256	264	272	280	287	295	303	311	319	326	334	342	350	358	365	373	381	389	396	404	412	420
75	152	160	168	176	184	192	200	208	216	224	232	240	248	256	264	272	279	287	295	303	311	319	327	335	343	351	359	367	375	383	391	399	407	415	423	431
76	156	164	172	180	189	197	205	213	221	230	238	246	254	263	271	279	287	295	304	312	320	328	336	344	353	361	369	377	385	394	402	410	418	426	435	443

Source: Adapted from Clinical Guidelines on the Identification, Evaluation, and Treatment of Overweight and Obesity in Adults: The Evidence Report.

National Heart Lung Blood Institute, www.nhlbi.nih.gov/guidelines/obesity/bmi_tbl.pdf

Complete
Wellness Seminar
Schedule One Today

I would like to bring a team to your church, school, or community to conduct a complete wellness seminar and help you know more. We can train people, in addition to your parish nurse, to implement an ongoing wellness program in your area. We can also demonstrate an exercise program you can use at home or wherever you are with little or no equipment. We begin slowly and work up to one hour per day, four days a week.

For a set of wellness materials that are available through CTS Family Press, please e-mail or write to me:

> Rev. Al Wingfield
> CTS Family Press
> 6600 North Clinton Street
> Fort Wayne, Indiana 46825
>
> Telephone: (260) 452-2106
>
> Fax: (260) 452-2121
>
> E-mail: al@alwingfield.com

A Special Seminar
for Families
The Christian Family Today

The *Christian Family Today* seminar was developed to help families from all walks of life take a closer look at what goes into healthy family relationships.

Whether you are experiencing difficulties with your spouse or children, or want to make a good relationship even better, this seminar will provide you with practical help that you can put to use right away. These are just a few of the questions that are discussed in *The Christian Family Today*:

- What role does "self-esteem" play in building a strong family?

- Will discipline damage my child's self-esteem?

- What causes marital breakdown, and what can be done to heal hurting relationships?

- When is divorce an option?

- What is the role of the church in building a strong family?

- Is forgiveness "for real"?

The seminar is led by the Reverend Albert B. Wingfield, author of *Marriage Is for Life—No Broken Promises, No Shattered Dreams*. Rev. Wingfield is a dynamic speaker who has the experience to back it up. Currently Vice President of Business Affairs at Concordia Theological Seminary in Fort Wayne, Indiana, Rev. Wingfield has also served in several Lutheran schools as teacher, dean of students, principal, headmaster, and superintendent.

The parents of six children, Rev. Wingfield and his wife Marge have, over the years, also opened their home to numerous foster children, international students, and elderly family members. They are now happy in their role as devoted grandparents.

There is much talk in the media about the "breakdown" in today's society and the decay of moral responsibility and values. What role can the church play in supporting and nurturing families? Rev. Wingfield will share his vision for implementing an "extended family" within the church and restoring the church to a more central position in building and upholding the family.

Additional guest speakers will bring their own experiences in dealing with a variety of family situations. You will learn what to expect in situations such as divorce or loss of a spouse or loved one; what to do with aging parents, troubled children, and teens; and how to ensure your family's financial future.

The seminar offers opportunities for discussion and role-playing as well as the traditional "lecture" style presentation. Ample time is provided for questions and interaction between speakers and seminar participants. Each seminar is unique, based on input from those who have registered.

Seminar topics include:

- Marriage
- Career Stress
- Children
- Aging Parents
- Single Parenting
- Schooling
- Teens
- Discipline
- Worship
- What should you expect from your church?
- What should your church expect from you?

For information on the date and location of the seminar nearest you, or to host a seminar at your church, contact:

Rev. Al Wingfield
CTS Family Press
6600 North Clinton Street
Fort Wayne, Indiana 46825

Telephone: (260) 452-2106

Fax: (260) 452-2121

E-mail: al@alwingfield.com